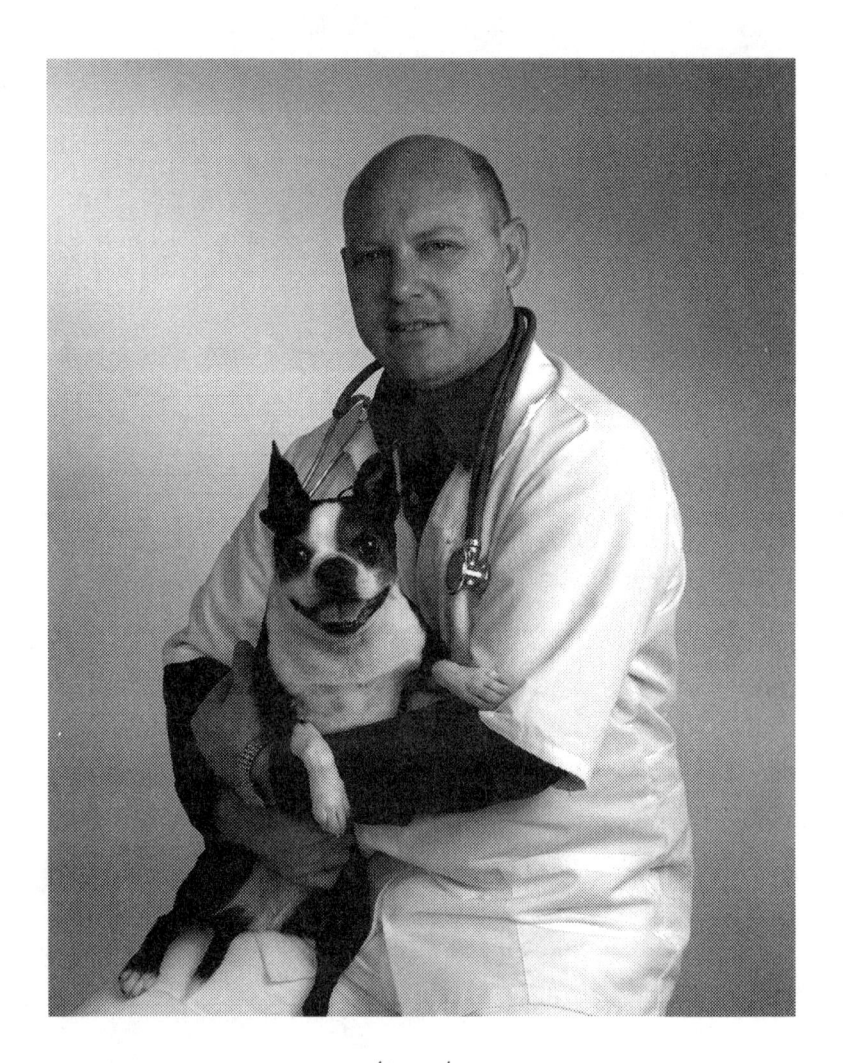

Alan and CC

Sleeping With Angels

A Veterinarian's Sacred Bond of Animal Companionship

By Alan Blain Cunningham

Sleeping With Angels: A Veterinarian's Sacred Bond of Animal Companionship

By Alan Blain Cunningham

Copyright © 2003 by Alan Blain Cunningham

ISBN 1-8881-0660-3
Library of Congress 2002116094

First Edition

All rights reserved. No part of this book may be reproduced or transmitted in any form or by any means, electronic or mechanical, including photocopying, recording, or by any information storage and retrieval system, without permission in writing from the copyright owner.

Cover design: Lea Taylor
Cover oil painting: James Raykovich

This book was printed in the United States of America.

Agreka LLC
800 360-5284
www.agreka.com

Dedication

This book is dedicated to my parents, family, supportive friends, and classmates at Oregon State University. Also it is devoted to the memory of my many animal companions whom I truly cherish and consider to be my angels, especially my beloved Pug.

Table of Contents

Introduction 9

Chapter 1
    One Step 13

Chapter 2
    Refiner's Fire 25

Chapter 3
    Transformation 39

Chapter 4
    A Second Chance 51

Chapter 5
    Freedom 71

Chapter 6
    Pug 87

Chapter 7
    Small Wonders 111

Chapter 8
    Farewell 125

Chapter 9
    Unconditional Love 139

Chapter 10
    A Breath Away 151

About the Author 167

Table of Illustrations

Pug and C.C. .... Cover
    By James Raykovich

One Step 12
    By Lisa Hull

Proud Pony 24
    By Lisa Hull

Jeanna 38
    By Lisa Hull

Bruiser 50
    By Lisa Hull

Stone Mountain 70
    By Lisa Hull

Pug 86
    By Lisa Hull

Rainbow Bridge 110
    By Lisa Hull

Rose 124
    By Lisa Hull

Legion of Angels 138
    By Lisa Hull and Brandon Rodriguez

Pug with Guardian Angel 150
    By Lisa Hull

Stepping Stone Journey .... 8 & 163
    By Lisa Hull

Paw Prints .... Throughout text
    By Lisa Hull

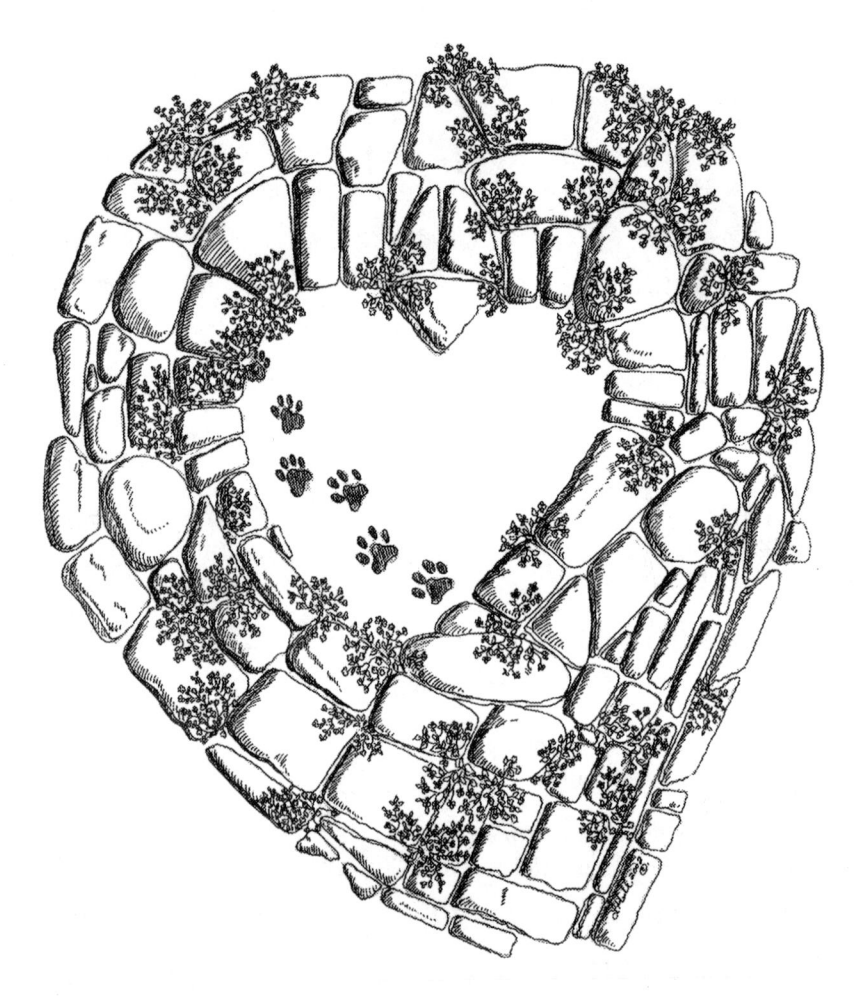

Stepping Stone Journey

Introduction

Throughout my life I have been fortunate to have animal companions. No matter what, I could always depend upon their loyal and unconditional friendship. I have learned to respect their precious existence and the obstacles they must endure. Their examples have given me strength and courage to face my own challenges. My animals are a source of comfort and safety to me. In fact, I value them as guardian angels.

During our journey on the bumpy road of life, we occasionally stumble along the way. Hopefully with determination, good friends (human or animal), and endurance, we can pick ourselves up and continue to reach our goals. One step at a time.

Relief from daily struggles can often be found in sleep. No greater trust can be gained than to have a true companion to share this time of sacred comfort with. I consider restful times with my animals as blessed moments to sleep with angels. A time of peace, comfort, tranquility, and hopeful strength.

As a lifelong student, I have come to know that science has limits, but love has no bounds. May this book *Sleeping With Angels* touch the stepping stones of your heart and provide you a tiny bit of comfort and strength. And may it also help you to realize that the distance between heaven and earth is a mere breath away.

Sincerely,

Alan Blain Cunningham

Sleeping With Angels

A Veterinarian's Sacred Bond of Animal Companionship

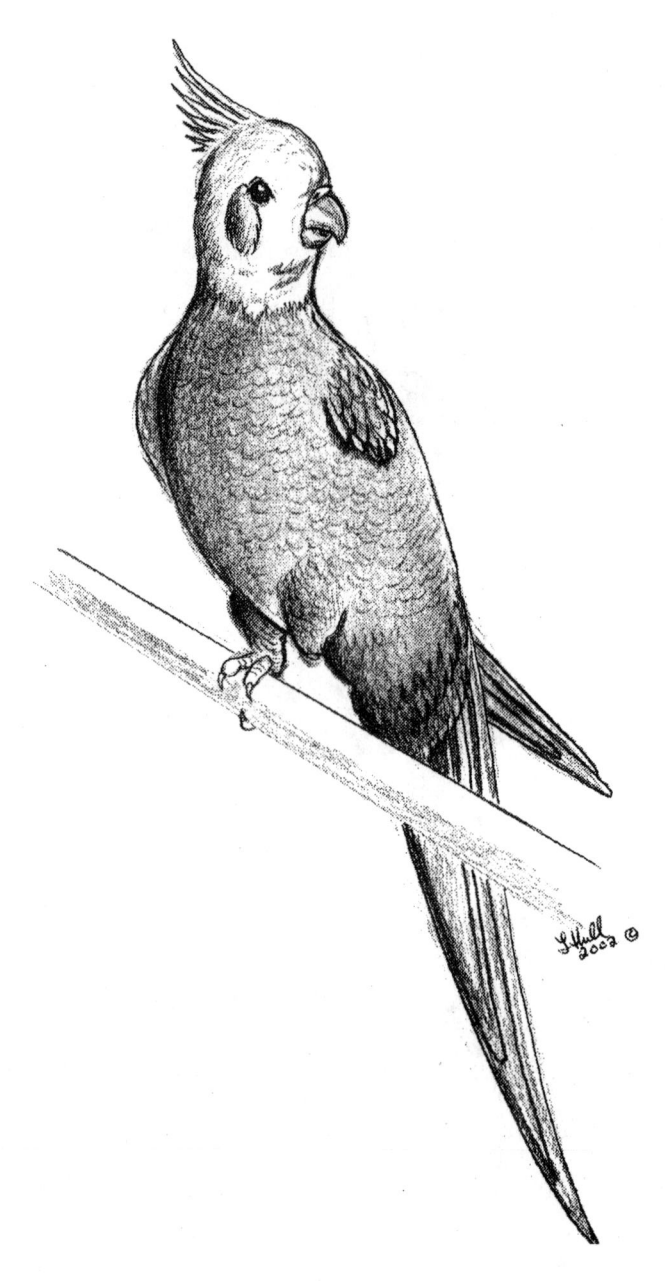

One Step

1
One Step

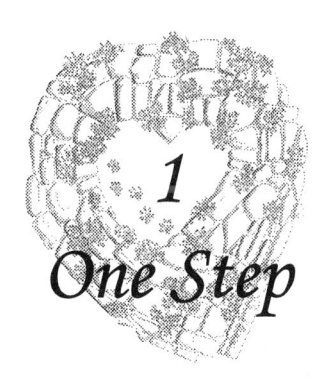

From an early age my parents taught me the importance of respecting all forms of life. When we would travel together as a family, Mom would excitedly direct our attention to the native wildlife. In rural areas she particularly pointed out newborn animals. Dad patiently helped me construct proper housing for the many pets I brought home.

My first pet was a stray female gray tabby cat. Mom, as was her nature, immediately named her. She called her China Doll because she was so fragile. I was about four years old when China Doll chose to stay at our home. My older brothers Jim and Bob each had pets — and I also wanted an animal companion. Jim owned a Quarter Horse named Rusty and a German Short Hair Pointer named Dusty. Bob raised rabbits. As big brothers often do, they took the opportunity to tease me.

"Only sissies have cats for pets," they taunted.

I suppose partly out of an attempt to please my brothers and also a childish curiosity, I decided to play a trick on China Doll. I picked her up and threw her as high as I possibly could, aiming for the roof of the house. She landed on her feet near the edge of the roof meowing at the top of her lungs. What a trick! Jubilantly I ran into the house to announce my achievement to mom.

"Come and see what I did, Mom — it's funny!"

She followed me outside.

"Isn't that funny," I laughed, pointing at China Doll.

Abruptly she replied, "Never, never do that again! How is she getting down?"

With a dejected and concerned voice I answered, "I don't know."

Mom demanded that I climb on her shoulders so I would be high enough to reach China Doll and bring her down from the roof.

"But Mom, I can't do that — I might fall," I trembled.

"Stand on my shoulders now!" she commanded, as she kneeled down.

Clumsily I climbed on her shoulders, frantically trying to keep my balance. Mom held tight to my legs. Surprised and trembling, I discovered that my hands reached the roof's edge. The height scared me. Mom, however, would not let me down.

"Now take hold of China Doll and lift her off the roof," she directed.

Slowly, awkwardly, I reached for my cat. With some encouragement on my part, and while I held onto the edge of the roof with my other hand, she allowed me to scruff her neck. And then she unexpectedly and painfully planted the claws of all four feet into my hand and arm. Finally, after what seemed like an eternity, she let loose of me, jumped away freely, and madly scurried off. My bleeding hand and arm were covered in scratches and bite marks. With little sympathy, Mom suggested that I should wash them, as she helped me to the ground.

"Never mistreat animals," she counseled.

"My mother taught me to never hurt or lie to

animals or to children," she concluded, "and I'm passing on the same advice to you."

Mom, by way of her mom, had taught me a granite lesson that I would always remember. To this day I have never again intentionally harmed an animal for the sake of curiosity, entertainment, or so called sportsmanship.

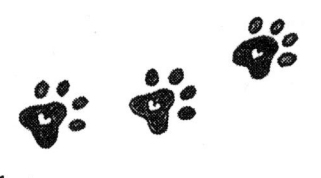

Several years later...

Grandma Gray had an assortment of chickens running freely in her yard. She lived alone and they were important company to her. They would nest in her coal shed, under her front porch, and wherever else one might imagine.

My Uncle Shorty owned an incubator and hatched many types of eggs. One summer day I discovered a nest of eggs in grandma's woodshed. Since they were unattended, I asked if I could take them to my uncle's to be incubated. Grandma agreed, my uncle obliged, and I enthusiastically delivered the eggs to be hatched.

The next day Aunt Lillian, mom's oldest sister, phoned and said that the eggs had blown up in the incubator. She laughed that I had brought them rotten eggs.

I quickly apologized and offered to help clean up the disaster.

She comforted, "That's okay. Listen, your Uncle Shorty has a pair of cockatiels he wants to give you. Would you like to have them?"

"You bet!" My youthful disappointment had turned to elation.

"Come over and Shorty will show you how to take care of them. Do you have a bird cage?"

"Yes, my brother Bob has one that I can use."

That afternoon Dad, Mom, and I drove to Uncle Shorty and Aunt Lillian's place. Uncle Shorty enthusiastically taught me about cockatiels. He explained that the pair I was getting were a breed called pieds. He added that normal grays, pearls, and albinos were other breed types.

"The pieds," he continued, "have white and gray bodies with yellow heads and orange cheeks. The males have a more intense orange." He said that they would probably live ten to twelve years and that I could teach them to talk, particularly the male.

"Have your dad help you make an outdoor confinement with a nesting box and next year they will breed. The nesting box must be deep enough to keep the young from getting out before they can fly. If the box isn't just right the birds won't breed, so let me give you this one," he offered.

"Thanks, Uncle Shorty," I replied. I hopefully looked at dad and he said that he would help me to build a proper cage for the cockatiels.

"Do you have names for them?" Aunt Lillian asked.

"Oh yes. The male is Tapioca and the female is Licorice." My niece Jan and nephews Troy and Ty had helped me choose the names.

"Let's go get them for you," Uncle Shorty interrupted. "Here's a package of bird seed until you can get some at the store."

I carried the bird cage into the large enclosure Uncle Shorty had built for the cockatiels and impressively watched as he easily caught them. They were like his pets.

Without hesitation Dad and my brother Bob helped me to begin construction on an outdoor cage for Tapioca and Licorice. In the meantime I kept them in the house. Sometimes I would let them out of their cage. Tapioca loved to perch on a shelf on Mom's china closet and gaze upon his reflection in the mirrored backing. He would spend countless hours perched on his throne admiring himself.

Some mornings he would wake me with his self-absorbing songs. Annoyed, I would throw a sock at him. Instead of it silencing him, he would either chirp more loudly or he would attack me boldly by landing on my shoulder and biting at my neck. Any other time Tapioca was very pleasant to be around and to handle.

Finally we completed the outdoor cage. The confinement was ten feet long, four feet wide, and eight feet tall. The structure was encased with one-inch chicken wire with a sturdy roof to protect the cockatiels from the sun, wind, rain, or snow. This was plenty of room for them to fly and to move about freely. Dad then mounted the nesting box high in the top center on the inside of the cage.

Sure enough, one year later Tapioca and Licorice nested and hatched out four eggs.

I learned many things: The incubation period is about twenty days. Newborns look like prehistoric pterodactyls with bald heads and orbital faces that are mostly eyes. Both parents diligently sit on the nest and take care of the hatchlings by forcing regurgitated feed into their hungry mouths.

As the newborns mature and grow feathers, they soon become agile enough to get out of the nesting box. The fledglings then perch on a small shelf located below the entrance hole of the box. With the encouragement of their parents, they carefully take the leap of faith and clumsily fly from perch to perch — each time, the distance getting further.

Daily, Tapioca and Licorice would steadfastly train their small flock of fledglings — back and forth, up and down they flew. At the end of each flight segment they would rest either on their perches or cling to the chicken wire cage.

One morning in late August, I checked on the new family of cockatiels. I was distressed to find one fledgling lying in the water container. Amazingly, he was still alive. But his left wing and left leg were completely amputated and it appeared as if they had been traumatically torn off.

My young niece Jan was with me at the time. "What are we going to do, Uncle?" she asked.

"I'm afraid the little thing is suffering," I replied. "I think it would be best if I destroyed him."

"Don't," she gasped, "he acts like he wants to live."

Carefully I lifted him out of the cold water and took him into the house. We quickly dried him off and cleaned his wounds. Fortunately, it didn't seem like much blood loss had occurred. Perhaps the cold water he landed in helped to constrict the blood vessels and slow the bleeding.

While Jan and I were conversing, Alamosa, my mixed breed Black Labrador, was sheepishly watching us. She had a particular curiosity for flying objects. For example, she would attack kites until she grounded them. To Alamosa, anything that was in the air must come down. I wondered if somehow she might have grabbed the cockatiel while he was clinging to the side of the cage. How she reached him through the chicken wire, I couldn't imagine. But I suspected Alamosa was more involved than she wanted us to know.

"I think we should place him back in his nest and let his parents take care of him," Jan said.

I cautiously agreed. I thought he would soon

Sleeping With Angels

die or that the parents would show no interest in him and he would eventually succumb to starvation. But Tapioca and Licorice continued to feed and care for him. To my pleasant surprise, he managed to grow and become stronger. While the other three youngsters became independent, this little one remained in the nesting box and continued to heal.

Eventually the Utah summer evolved into early autumn. Mom reminded, "It's getting chilly now, perhaps we should bring One Step into the house."

I looked at Mom and realized that she had given him a name.

"Oh yes," she responded. "I have all the babies named."

Sometimes, even if my animals already had names, Mom would give them one of her own. As a result, many of my animals answered to two names. We unanimously agreed that One Step, our one-legged little cockatiel, was an appropriate name.

The parents and two of the siblings would remain outside with a heat lamp turned on in the cage when the weather eventually turned cold. Otherwise One Step and his sister, who mom named

Thumbelina because of her tiny size, would be transferred into the house.

Unfortunately Thumbelina died shortly after the move. But One Step continued to thrive. He would maneuver in his environment using his beak and right foot to grasp his perch or the side of his cage. Cleverly he would also use his beak to open the door to his enclosure and balance himself upon its threshold.

Ever so slowly, little by little, step by step — with the courage and heart of a giant — One Step began to master his tiny world. His wholehearted determination both impressed and inspired me.

My nephews Troy and Ty continually talked to One Step and before long he responded and entertained us with imitations of "pretty bird," "hello," the charge whistle, and the cat call whistle. He even copied the ambulance siren, which the little guy must have taught himself since none of us made that annoying sound to him.

Each morning, with only one leg and one wing, One Step would enthusiastically perch upon his open door and begin to sing as if to herald, "Good morning beautiful world, isn't it great to be alive!"

Sleeping With Angels

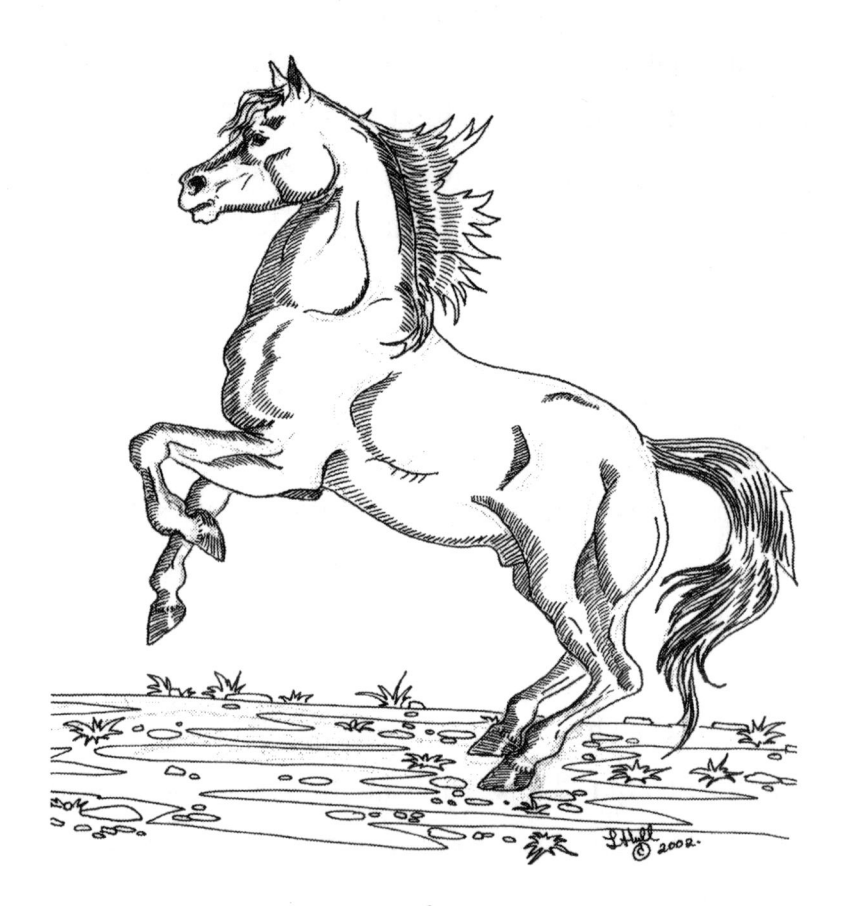

Proud Pony

2
Refiner's Fire

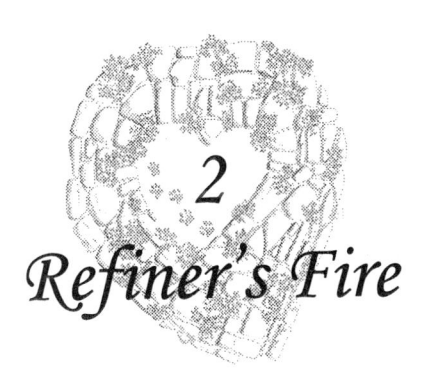

In 1982, at the age of twenty-six, a lifetime dream came true. I was accepted into the Colorado State University School of Veterinary Medicine. I had already obtained my Bachelor of Science in Animal Science from Brigham Young University and was ready to fulfill my long awaited goal. For as long as I could remember, veterinary medicine was the profession I wanted. Since there are relatively few veterinary schools in the United States, getting accepted is difficult. But I had worked hard and was one of the lucky few.

My entire energy was focused on excelling in the veterinary school. I realized the training would be rigorous and difficult. In order to commit as much time and energy as possible to school, I decided to live on campus in the dorm, closer to my classes. Also I decided to leave my car at home in Utah so that I would not be tempted to engage in too many extracurricular activities.

My parents accompanied me to Ft. Collins where the school was located and repeatedly expressed how proud they were of me. I was so excited to begin my lifetime ambition that I hardly realized when they left.

The first day of classes were filled with anticipation and excitement. The faculty members introduced themselves and congratulated us upon being an elite group of select students embarking upon an honorable profession.

The entire freshman class, one hundred forty students strong, was a various assortment of ages, personalities, and professional aspirations. The gender ratio consisted of approximately sixty percent male and forty percent female. I was impressed and intrigued to discover that a mother and son were included as my classmates.

Our class advisor, we discovered, would also be our anatomy and histology professor. Remarkably brilliant, he mastered the first names of the entire class within a few days. I also noticed he was arrogant, obnoxious, and vulgar.

He introduced the courses for the first semester, boasting that most of our time would be spent with him since he was the lead coordinator for functional anatomy, which consisted of physiology, neurology, histology, and anatomy. The remaining classes included bacteriology, virology, mycology, and animal breeds.

From day one I struggled with one particular class — functional anatomy. Not only did I dislike the instructor and his methods, but the conglomerate class consisted of too much material for me.

The first functional anatomy exam was a disaster. I miserably failed.

Afterwards I committed to simply work harder. I would carry a sack lunch to school and study while I ate, or arise earlier in the morning, and study later at night. Unfortunately this technique only made me tired and hungry and less able to concentrate effectively.

Most of the semester was laboriously monopolized with painstakingly repetitious study of processed and fresh animal cadavers; and memorization of bones, muscles, nerves, vessels, tendons, ligaments, insertions, origins, on and on. The smell of the embalming formaldehyde was sickening to me. I longed to work with live animals.

Fortunately the opportunity arrived when we started to learn about nerve blocks on horse legs.

Next to the spacious anatomy lab were some stalls with live horses for us to palpate the anatomical landmarks and sites for injecting local anesthetics. I became especially fond of one obstinate and proud pony. Although he was difficult to handle sometimes, he was reasonable if treated patiently. Oftentimes, when no one else was around, I would visit him just for the companionship of a live animal.

All too soon we had another anatomy exam impending, with emphasis on the horse legs. Actually the anatomy of a horse's leg is spectacular. They are such powerful appendages and yet so weak, especially with all the lameness problems and the foot ailments. And I could never fully appreciate the "stay" apparatus that allowed the graceful athletic giants to stand while sleeping.

Because the preserved horse cadavers were

so restrictively expensive, we often used freshly amputated horse legs to study. The heat of early autumn afternoons became intolerably uncomfortable in the huge anatomy lab. So the large outside service doors leading to the enormous room were propped open. We were grateful for the gentle afternoon breeze flowing through the area.

Unfortunately, flies also followed. After one or two days, the fresh meat of the horse carcasses became putrid, maggot infested, and nearly unbearable to dissect. Even though the body parts were stored in refrigeration when not being examined, they still became rancid fairly quickly.

The ominous day for the equine anatomy exam finally arrived. With a great deal of distress I felt less prepared for this exam than any other. Reluctantly I entered the lab with half of my other classmates. The vast space was carefully arranged with tagged animal parts waiting to be identified. Aghast, I spotted my tagged and dissected pony friend hanging on meat hooks from the ceiling.

The foundation seemed to crumble beneath me and no matter how hard I tried, I could not regain my focus or think clearly. The allotted test time passed in a haze. Most of my test answers were wrong or left blank. I could not bring myself to get close to the destroyed pony.

I had failed another anatomy exam. More importantly, I felt like I had lost a good and honest friend in the pony.

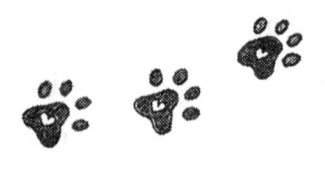

Thanksgiving vacation arrived. I had eagerly anticipated the return home to my family and animals, not to mention a brief escape from veterinary school. Back home, I wrestled with my experiences at school. Finally I decided that perhaps the independence of having my car at school would help relieve some of the pressure. Dad volunteered to help me drive back to Ft. Collins, then he planned to fly home. He was trying to give me support.

The time arrived to take Dad to the Denver Airport. As we were waiting for his plane I watched him. Something was wrong. He would unsteadily stand and then ever so slightly tip forward. Almost unknowingly, he seemed to quickly right himself. Later on I learned that he was exhibiting intention tremors or neurological deficits to the coordination center of his brain. Because Dad had previously undergone open heart bypass surgery, I feared that he was either having more heart problems or possibly a stroke.

"Are you okay, Dad?" I asked as he prepared to board the plane.

"I'm just fine, son," he smiled.

As he shook my hand goodbye, tears welled up in his eyes and then quickly he gathered himself and said goodbye.

"Thanks Dad," I offered as I sadly waved back.

After that my thoughts seemed to focus on Dad, home, family, and my animals. In truth, veterinary school had become a nightmare for me. I did not feel elite or proud. Needless to say, I failed my first semester. With the enthusiasm and excitement I had started out the semester, the last thing I imagined was to end the sixteen weeks at such an extremely low level. Possibly the lowest point of my life up to that time.

After driving home for the holidays, I purchased a round trip airline ticket and nervously traveled back to Ft. Collins. Because of formalities I was allowed to retake the functional anatomy final during Christmas break. Unfortunately I failed the exam. The admissions committee interviewed me and voted four to one not to allow me to come back and rejoin the next year's class.

The teacher I disliked so much was on the committee. He said, "You're a twenty mile an hour person in a fifty mile an hour speed zone. You don't belong here."

My dignified response, "Yeah, well you're a jerk too."

To this day, I recall this statement as being the most exhilarating event of my entire CSU experience.

Afterwards, I phoned my parents. I informed them of the outcome.

They said, "We're coming to take you home."

Dad and Mom drove all night from American Fork, Utah, to Ft. Collins, Colorado, without sleep in order to be with me in my time of need. In the meantime a true friend and classmate, Ron Carsten, kept me company. Thank you Ron.

Dad and Mom arrived early that cold December morning. Initially they were so exhausted they fell asleep on my motel bed. When they awoke we had a refreshing breakfast and then started the journey back home.

Mom asked me, "Is it possible some of the teachers at the school do not feel about animals the way you do?"

I thought about her question for several minutes. "Mom, it seems to be nothing but a business to a few of the teachers."

Mom then told me about a song Ruthann had sung to her called "Beans and Beets." Ruthann was my brother Bob's youngest daughter. She was quite a little character even at the age of three. I could picture her performing her song and the depiction made me chuckle. For the first time in several months I was able to honestly and freely laugh.

I felt as if a huge weight had been lifted from my shoulders. I was returning to my home, a place where I was valued and accepted, a place where I could recover a sense of who I was. And, of course, there were my precious animals.

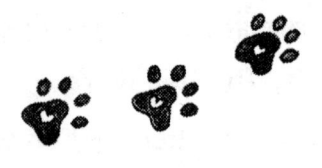

Looking back, I'm glad for the unexpected detour in my life from veterinary school because it allowed me to reassess and more fully appreciate an experience I had when I was just nineteen.

As I was growing up in the Mormon Church I had begrudged the idea of being expected to serve as a missionary for my religion when I turned of age. My answer to such a calling was a contrite "no." At the time, my main goal was to get into veterinary school and I did not want to lose two years to missionary service

One night, just before turning nineteen, I dreamed that the old church building where I attended services was on fire. This was especially significant to me since I worked as a custodian at that building in real life. In my dream the flames were unquenchable. Desperately I called for the surrounding neighbors to help me control the roaring fire. They would hook up their hoses to outdoor faucets and bring them to me.

But instead of helping me spray the fire, they

would just lay the hoses with running water at my feet. Exhausted, I fell into tears knowing that I could not extinguish the fire by myself. As my tears subsided I looked up and beheld a new, beautiful church building standing in place of the old.

The next morning I changed my mind about serving a mission and decided that I would go. I didn't fully understand my dream. I felt that many people could help and support me, but as far as serving a mission — I had to do that myself. And if I did, I would somehow return a better person.

Two weeks into my mission experience my parents wrote and informed me that the church building we attended had burned down. I replied and described to them how it burned, and where it started. I said that when the firemen sprayed water on it, it was more like gasoline than water because the building quickly disintegrated. And I told them of my dream. A few days later my parents wrote back and said that my dream was exactly like it happened.

Two years later when I returned home from my mission, a beautiful new building was standing in place of the old. Mom and I worked as custodians of the new structure for several years.

My brief experience at Colorado State University had been like my dream — disintegrating in unquenchable flames. I had felt completely and helplessly destroyed at the time. In fact, I felt as if God had forsaken me.

But now I realize that because of the experience, I am a better and stronger person, and a more committed veterinarian.

Footprints in the Sand

One night a man had a dream. He dreamed he was walking along the beach with the Lord. Across the sky flashed scenes from his life. For each scene, he noticed two sets of footprints in the sand; one belonging to him, and the other to the Lord.

When the last scene flashed before him, he looked back at the footprints and noticed that many times along the path there was only one set of footprints in the sand. He also noticed that this happened during the lowest and saddest times in his life.

This really bothered him, so he questioned the Lord, "Lord, you said that once I decided to follow you, you would walk with me all the way, but I noticed that during the most troublesome times of my life, there was only one set of footprints. I don't understand why. When I needed you the most, you deserted me."

The Lord replied, "My precious, precious child, I love you and would never leave you. During your times of trial and suffering, when you see only one set of footprints, it was then that I carried you."

Author Unknown

Sleeping With Angels

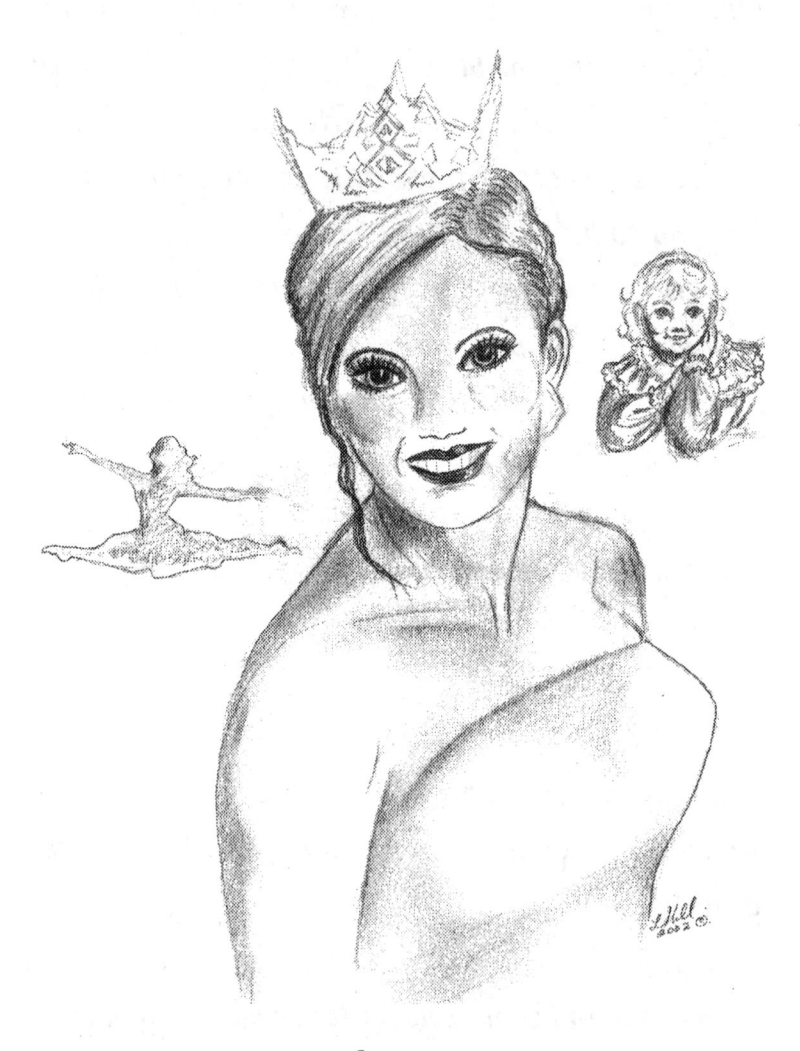

Jeanna

3
Transformation

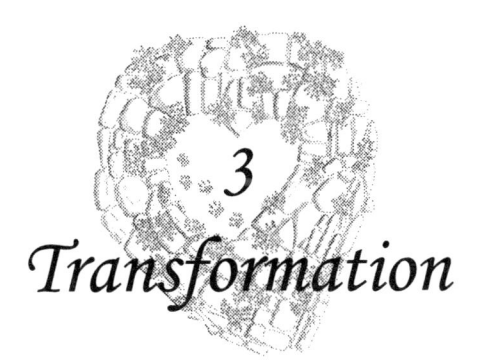

Returning home after failing in veterinary school was a double-edged sword. I was remorseful that I had disappointed everyone, including myself. And I was angry, depressed, felt rejected and was embarrassed. At times I thought of myself as completely worthless. On the other hand, I was home and in the surroundings that I loved most, with my family and animals. As I viewed it, life could only get better.

Unfortunately, regaining my self worth was difficult. Completing simple tasks such as washing the car seemed like a notable accomplishment for me. One dreary January morning, while cleaning the basement, my oldest brother Jim and his youngest daughter Jeanna visited. He addressed me with a cheerful "Hello, doctor." I looked up and smiled and was grateful for the sincere and uplifting greeting.

My niece Jeanna was just learning to walk. And for a moment I stepped out of my own despair long enough to observe her. She would clumsily proceed a few steps and then stumble. When she fell, she would briefly whimper from the insulting pain. But then with renewed determination she would pick herself up and move ahead a few more steps until she fell again. This pattern persisted until Jim gathered her up in his arms.

Each time she stumbled and fell I would hopefully and silently encourage "get back up little girl, you can do it." Eventually she learned to walk — one step at a time.

Through the years I have witnessed Jeanna transform from an awkward toddler into a national champion dancer and beauty queen. I also proudly watched as she carried the torch for the 2002 Winter Olympics in Salt Lake City. Little does she realize the brave example of courage and perseverance that she provided for me when she was a young girl.

"Just get back up, you can do it."

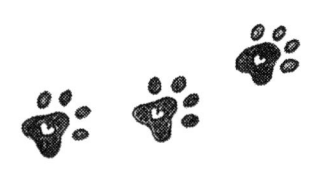

A few weeks later my father relayed some promising information to me. While receiving a health exam at the hospital from the pulmonary physician, he learned that the respiratory care department was seeking students for on the job training to become respiratory therapists.

"The doctor gave me a phone number for you to call," he offered.

I was excited but at the same time hesitant about failure. "Just get back up," an inner voice encouraged, "You can do it."

With some uncertainty I dialed the number. A pleasant voice answered, "Utah Valley Hospital, respiratory care, how can I help you?"

"Hi, this is Alan Cunningham, I'm interested in the respiratory therapy training program."

"I'm sorry," she politely informed, "the class is full. We have all the students we need. I will write down your name, however, and if we have any changes I will call you. What is your phone number, please?"

Disappointed, I gave her the number and said "Thank you."

"You're welcome, and goodbye," she professionally acknowledged.

The following week the same lady called. "Hi, this is Diane. I talked with you last week about the respiratory therapy program. One of the students has withdrawn from the class due to health problems. Are you still interested?" she asked.

"Yes! I answered.

"Classes start tomorrow," she continued. "I apologize for the late notice but I just found out about the opening myself. Can you be here in the respiratory classroom tomorrow from eight a.m. to five p.m?"

"Yes, of course."

"Thank you, and see you tomorrow, Alan."

I arrived the next morning with concern and excitement. Bob Guenter and Charles Lyons were our instructors — and I liked them. The class consisted of five students: Holly, Janet, Dean, Kim, and myself. We were all about the same age and all college graduates in a science field.

Although the class work was intense, the atmosphere was conducive to learning. Since the hospital badly needed respiratory therapists, we were made to feel important, useful, and wanted.

To my own comfort no one would be allowed to fail or to be made a sacrificial token in order to make the program appear more accredited.

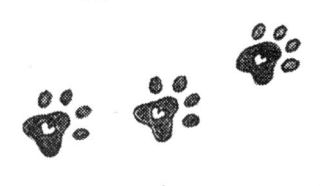

Following one month of rigorous training we were allowed to begin working with the hospital patients. I recall a beautiful dark-haired little girl about three years old. When I approached her, she brightened with a huge smile. She eagerly watched me through the side rails of her bed. I observed that she had a tracheostomy, the artificial opening into her throat so that she could breathe. Sadly, I had been informed that her father had abused her and damaged her face so badly that she could not breathe adequately through her nose and mouth. Thus the tracheostomy tube.

I wondered how she could be so trusting and open to me after being mistreated by an adult male. She continued to follow me with her hopeful large eyes and cherubic broad smile. My heart melted and I tenderly picked her up and hugged her. Although she could not talk because of the trach tube, she responded with an ever widening grin.

What a commanding lesson on not giving up on life and becoming bitter, I reminded myself, "Get up, you can do it."

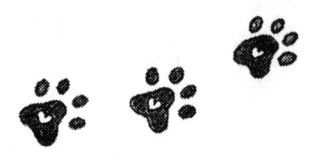

Another patient, Pam, who was about forty years old, was hospitalized in the psychiatric ward for suicide attempts. She also had asthma and required frequent breathing treatments. I was assigned to provide her respiratory care every four hours throughout the day.

"Hi," I announced, "I'm with respiratory. May I give you a breathing treatment?"

She did not respond. Instead she cautiously followed me with mistrusting eyes.

"Let me give you this treatment. I'll sit next to you while you take it, is that okay?"

Still Pam did not respond other than to open her hand when I offered her the nebulizer. A few minutes later she looked around and quietly probed, "Do you have a gun?"

"No," I answered, taken aback and alarmed.

"I want to shoot myself."

Not knowing what to say, I quietly turned to leave, then offered to see her again in four hours.

"If I'm still alive," she threatened.

Four hours later, still unsettled by my initial encounter with Pam, I hesitantly returned to her room. This time she seemed more cheerful and not as cautious towards me. I was relieved.

"How are you?" she asked.

"Fine thanks," I returned.

She apologized about that morning. With some reserve I answered, "That's okay."

"Tell me about yourself. You seem like a nice guy," she continued.

Again I was somewhat hesitant. "I like animals and would like to become a veterinarian."

"Oh really," she easily responded. As if to read my mind she then asked, "What kind of animals do you have?"

"Dogs, cats, chickens, and a cockatiel," I offered.

"What is the cockatiel's name?"

"His name is One Step."

"Why did you name him that?"

While Pam took her breathing treatment, I revealed One Step's story. Afterwards she expressed that she would like to meet him.

"Perhaps I can arrange to bring him by if the nurse will permit it. I have tomorrow off from work." Fortunately, the nurse readily gave me permission.

The next afternoon One Step and I visited Pam. She was lying in bed. "I've been looking forward to your visit. What a beautiful bird," she exclaimed.

One Step responded with the cat call whistle. Pam giggled. "May I hold him? . . .I will be very gentle."

"Yes, you may," I allowed. I was secretly skeptical that she might harm him. Slowly I lifted One Step from his cage and offered him to Pam to hold.

"I'll place him right here by my arm," she reassured me.

Pam had beautiful thick, dark red hair that draped across her shoulder. One Step immediately proceeded to preen it. He would carefully take a few strands and tenderly run it through his beak as if cleaning her hair. Quietly she watched.

"This is the most contented I've felt for a long time," she expressed. Pam seemed to enjoy One Step's companionship and marveled at his abilities since he only had one wing and one leg. In return One Step seemed to thrive on the attention and freely offered his entire repertoire of whistles, songs, and phrases.

For the first time since meeting Pam, I watched her face shine with happiness. And I hoped the thought of killing herself had vanished. Shortly afterwards she was released from the hospital and returned to work as a registered nurse.

Partially as a result of One Step, Pam and I became good friends. And even more importantly, she was able to resume a functional life.

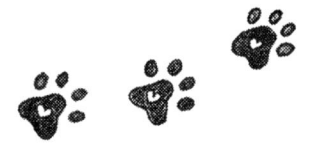

One year had elapsed since leaving veterinary school and beginning work as a respiratory therapist. Whenever I began to doubt or feel sorry for myself, all I had to do was look at the patients I was caring for. Many of them struggled simply to breathe. I soon realized how extremely fortunate I was.

Thankfully, success as a respiratory therapist helped me to start believing in myself again. I passed the national board exams to become a registered respiratory therapist. Also I completed a master's degree in respiratory health care science at Brigham Young University. Daringly, I even ran a marathon and parachuted from a plane.

Yet I still yearned to become a veterinarian and decided to enroll in classes more directed towards veterinary medicine. Since I experienced difficulty in functional anatomy while at Colorado State University, I decided to pursue instruction in that area. In the autumn of 1984 I was accepted into the biology doctorate program at Utah State University in Logan, Utah. With the guidance of LeGrande Ellis, my graduate advisor, I obtained a Ph.D. in physiology three years later.

During my final year at USU I applied to veterinary school at Oregon State University in Corvallis, Oregon. Dad and Mom accompanied me to the admissions interview that spring. On the way, I was tempted to turn around and go back home.

"Pull yourself up, you can do it," an inner voice again persuaded.

A couple months later I received a letter from OSU stating that the entering class had been selected, and that I was an alternate. Although the news was disappointing, it was not a total rejection. Some hope of acceptance remained.

Shortly afterwards a notice arrived from OSU. They informed me that one of the Utah students had accepted a position at another veterinary school. As a result, a seat had become available to me as an alternate.

Without hesitation, I replied, "I'll be there."

I had been given a second chance to reach my lifetime dream.

Sleeping With Angels

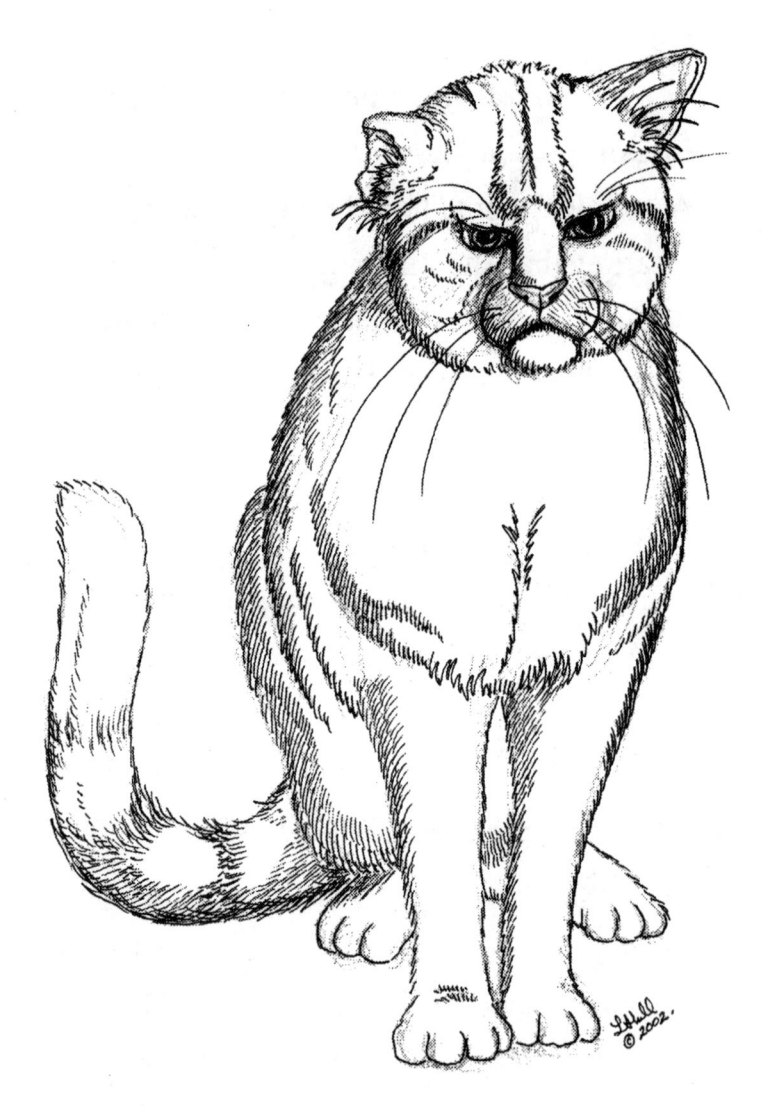

Bruiser

4
A Second Chance

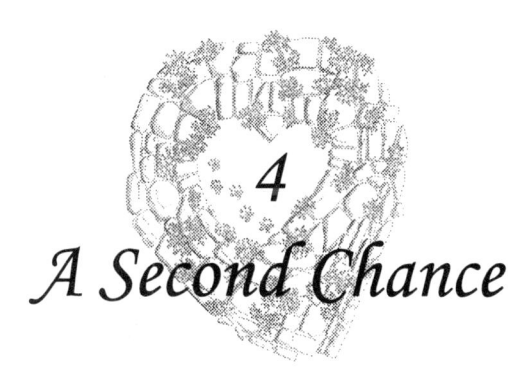

In the autumn of 1987 my lifetime dream of becoming a veterinarian was rekindled. I joined the entering Class of 1991 at the Oregon State University School of Veterinary Medicine in Corvallis, Oregon.

Corvallis is located nearby the coast of the Pacific Northwest and is beautifully nestled in a lush green, wooded area. I lived in a mobile home park off campus next to a lumber mill. In the late summer and early autumn the air was fragrant with freshly milled logs, and the blackberry bushes were plentiful with sweet, succulent fruit. The atmosphere and surrounding landscape seemed pleasant and inviting to me. Somehow I sensed that my second chance at veterinary school would be successful.

Again the faculty welcomed us as a prestigious group of students. The class of thirty-six consisted of eighteen men and eighteen women. Because we were a relatively small group, we quickly became like a family. Not only would we spend long strenuous days together in the classroom and labs, we also joined together in extracurricular activities such as sports, movies, and picnics. And although school in itself was extremely demanding, we did manage to find some time for fun.

Towards the end of our freshman year the class planned to take a couple hours break in the afternoon and play volleyball at the school's fitness center. If nothing else, we managed to relieve some tension and to have a good time.

As we were ending our activity one day, I leaped up to slam the volleyball across the net. While coming down I felt a tremendous strain in my lower back. I hobbled to the side of the court to wait out the rest of the match and decided I had probably pulled or strained a muscle.

Being thirty-one years of age, I was one of the older class members. I had also prematurely lost most of my hair to male pattern baldness. Consequently, I was the target for many good-natured "old man" comments.

"What's wrong, old man, the women wearing you out?"

"Hell, I can just stand here and watch your body parts fall off even as we speak," another added.

"Just give me a minute and I'll beat the sh— out of the entire bunch of you," I jokingly warned.

The game shortly ended and I limped back to school with the rest of my classmates.

"My grandma could beat you in a foot race, old man," a classmate ridiculed with a smile.

"Yeah, I'll take you, and your mama, and your grandma all on," I challenged.

The remainder of the afternoon became painfully and agonizingly slow. "If I can just hold out until the day is over then I can lie down, get some rest, and feel better by the morning," — I hoped. But no matter how I positioned myself — standing, lying, sitting — the persistent pain was nearly unbearable.

The next day, after a restless night of sleep, I arrived late to school and had to drag myself into class. By then my classmates were more sympathetic and supportive and they encouraged me to seek medical help at the school's health center.

That afternoon I checked into the center. The attending physician announced we should take some x-rays. The results indicated nothing abnormal. "Perhaps you have pulled or strained a deep muscle," he suggested. "Let me prescribe some pain medication and muscle relaxants for you."

Before retiring that night, I took the prescribed medication and fell into a fitful sleep of hallucinogenic dreams. "This is no good," I worried. "If I take the medications, I certainly won't be able to concentrate on my class work." On the other hand, I soon discovered that if I didn't use the drugs, I would become nauseously painful and still unable to study effectively.

"Just tough it out," I pledged to myself. "Freshman year is nearly over. You can do it. Once summer break arrives, you can return home and relax. Perhaps it's just stress."

Try as I may, I was only getting worse. We were nearing finals and I had recently failed a pathology midterm. My right leg started to become numb and I could not feel my foot. I returned to the university medical doctor and told him of my symptoms. He referred me to a neurosurgeon. I readily accepted and visited him for consultation a few days later.

The neurosurgeon carefully examined me and concluded that I had herniated a disc in my lower back. He informed me that sometimes the cushioned contents of the discs in between the vertebrae can rupture. He indicated that the resulting pressure from the protruding disc on the nerve roots can lead to severe, constant pain, and numbness to the affected leg and foot.

"In order to more accurately diagnose the problem we need to perform a myelogram," he continued. "This means that we inject dye into your spinal column. Then we take fluoroscopic x-rays of your spine to see if there are any areas where there is a thinning or complete obliteration of the dye column. This indicates a ruptured disc," he informed. "We can perform the procedure tomorrow."

"The sooner the better," I said.

The myelogram detected a large area of ruptured disc in my lower back. "Just as expected," the doctor commented. "I'm surprised that you're still going to school. In fact, I'm amazed that you can even walk. Perhaps the best and quickest treatment would be to surgically remove the ruptured disc material so we can get you back on your feet without pain.

Again I reiterated, "The sooner the better."

"In the meantime, you must lie very still on your back," he cautioned. "We punctured your spinal cord to inject the dye and now it needs time to heal."

I remained quietly in the hospital bed that afternoon waiting impatiently to be released.

I had already missed a couple days of school and was severely behind in my class work. I was failing pathology. I figured the sooner I had the surgery, the quicker I could continue on with classes.

Suddenly the events of Colorado State haunted my mind. I did not want to experience that nightmare again.

"I must get back to school," I insisted to the nurse.

She explained, "Normally we require our patients to rest longer," but when I didn't relent, she said she would allow me to leave.

I slowly hobbled out of the hospital. Initially, I had planned on returning to school for the remainder of the afternoon classes. However, I soon discovered that I felt too badly and instead drove myself home. I felt miserable physically and emotionally. Not only did my right leg hurt, but now I had a pounding headache. I was failing school and I had no medical insurance. That night was insufferable.

The next morning I simply gave up. I forced myself to school and requested to speak with Dr. Hutton, the assistant dean in charge of admissions. Fortunately he was there and invited me into his office. I explained that I had been diagnosed with a herniated disc in my lower spine and that the resulting pain in my leg and head was unbearable.

"I want to quit," I anguished. "I can't continue like this."

Thankfully he was understanding and encouraged me to take care of my physical needs. "We will figure something out later," he added.

By this time the pain, especially in my head, was so severe that I could barely stand. A few classmates accompanied me to the emergency room at the Corvallis Good Samaritan Hospital. I informed the emergency physician that I had a myelogram to detect a herniated disc the day before and since then had been burdened with an extreme headache.

"Let me call your doctor," he suggested.

Shortly afterwards he returned. He explained that sometimes as a result of the diagnostic procedure, fluid will leak from the spine at the injection site. "The imbalance of fluids," he continued, "changes pressures on the brain and creates severe headaches. We need to transfer you to anesthesiology immediately," he ordered.

The anesthesiologist related that he would draw some blood from my arm and inject it into my spine. He commented that this would form a blood patch or clot over the puncture site in my spinal column and allow the fluid pressures to return to normal.

"We must keep you in the hospital, however, until you feel better."

A Second Chance

Fortunately the procedure was a success, and my headache cured. The next day surgery was performed to remove the herniated disc and that too was a success. At last I was mercifully free of pain.

When I awoke, Mom, Dad, and my brother Bob were waiting to visit me. My father, bless his heart, was now in a wheelchair, but was determined to come and help bring me home. Since my brother had to leave before I was discharged, Uncle Jay, and Mom's twin sister Aunt Bareen, were also there to help take me home.

Throughout the day classmates filed into my room to visit and to give me encouragement. I would remain in the hospital a couple of days and then return home. In the meantime my parents handled the billing arrangements.

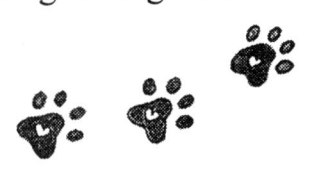

I departed from Corvallis fearing that my future in veterinary school had ended. If nothing else, I thought, at least I had made some special friends and would dearly miss them.

A few days after arriving home to Utah, a letter arrived from Dr. Hutton. He stated that the professors had agreed to let me take my finals during the summer break as soon as I had healed. He added that if I failed any of the exams, I would be dismissed from veterinary school. Then he closed with, "Good luck."

Apparently my classmates had been informed of my predicament. A large packet arrived with the class notes for the quarter. In it was a letter: "We have chosen the best notes of the class for each subject area and highlighted the areas for you to concentrate on in your studies. Several classmates that are remaining on campus through the summer have agreed to tutor you when you return to take the finals. Good luck, old man!"

How could I fail with that much genuine support? Immediately I was determined to succeed. I left veterinary school in late May and was required by the doctor to recuperate for six weeks.

Sophomore year would start in early September. I eagerly calculated my schedule to begin taking finals at the end of July and throughout August. I relayed my time schedule to all the teachers involved and started anxiously to prepare for the tests.

When I arrived at Oregon State University, my classmates were excited to review with me. One by one, step by step, I successfully passed all of the exams. Just one day before sophomore year started, I received the final passing grade for pathology class.

Graciously and thankfully to my wonderful classmates, I was given yet another second chance to pursue my dream.

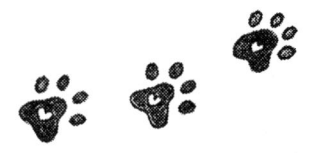

While I was at OSU taking finals, Dad's condition worsened. He had been diagnosed with a degenerative brain lesion to the coordination center of his brain. The pathology was identified as chronic pontine cerebellar dysplasia. Dad's speech and swallowing became severely compromised. In addition, he couldn't walk and had to use a wheelchair. In order to help him obtain the nourishment he needed, the doctor placed a gastrostomy feeding tube directly into his stomach. This way Mom could more easily support his diet with Ensure, a high caloric liquid food supplement.

Often I worried if I would see Dad alive again when I left home for long periods of time. Therefore, after finishing my exams, I quickly returned home.

Unfortunately I had to leave the next day to begin sophomore year at Washington State University Veterinary School in Pullman, Washington. And although I was excited and relieved to continue with my wonderful classmates, I was also concerned about Dad's health. But no matter his needs, he always gave me one hundred percent support in my goals, and wished me well as I left.

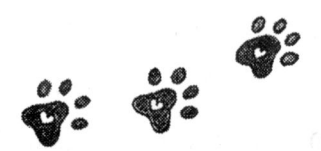

When I arrived at Washington State University, I was greeted with hugs and handshakes from my classmates. And, oh yes, a few "old man" comments.

At the time, OSU was a relatively new and non-accredited veterinary school without complete facilities for all the necessary training that we needed. Therefore the second and most of our third year of school were spent at WSU, which was a more fully accredited veterinary university with complete teaching facilities. We teamed with sixty-four students at WSU to become a combined class of one hundred members.

During junior year, the OSU students began clinical rotation during winter semester. The WSU students continued in class work. Our clinical rotations usually consisted of three or four students and an advisor, and lasted about two weeks each.

While in small animal medicine rotation, we were routinely assigned nighttime critical care shifts. During the shift we would administer prescribed treatments and medications that the attending veterinarians had ordered. Also we would monitor the hospitalized animals.

One night shift I was introduced to a tattered, stray tomcat in critical care. He had gotten caught in the fan belt of a car. During cold weather, cats often rest on car engines to keep warm. Sadly, when the engine is started, the unsuspecting cat becomes severely harmed and often killed.

This battle-scarred, orange tabby cat, although

severely injured, had managed to live. He looked like he had just finished a ten round heavyweight boxing match. His eyes were swollen shut, his face bruised and cut, and one ear was missing. Also the skin on his right front leg was stripped away, exposing his muscles and tendons.

In spite of his trauma, the war torn cat patiently persevered. He willingly allowed me to treat him and then would either eat or go back to sleep. "What a trooper," I thought, "he just goes on in life without showing the slightest complaint. I like this guy."

Several days passed. My new tabby friend was moved from critical care to a boarding area. I kept an eye on him. "What's his fate?" I asked our advisor.

She said that a good Samaritan had rescued him and brought him in. She was hopeful they could find a home for him, but she cautiously added that he was a carrier of feline aids. "Since it is a contagious viral disease to other cats, we might have a hard time placing him. Perhaps he will be euthanized and considered a teaching or research project."

"May I take him?" I asked.

She shrugged, "If you want to."

"Yes, I do."

At that moment I named him Bruiser. He was tough, non-complaining, and certainly looked the part.

That night I took Bruiser home from the teaching hospital. We had already become friends but we continued to bond. He allowed me to change the dressing on his right front leg daily. Slowly the wounds began to heal and to granulate in. I was pleased to have a companion. I already had fish, but they didn't really count as pets to me.

For some reason, possibly because of his wanderlust lifestyle, Bruiser would not use the litter box. Instead he regularly urinated and defecated on or under my bed. As a result I occasionally allowed him outside to do his business. One night in late January, I let him out. Since it was too cold to stay with him, I briefly hurried back into my apartment and determined to let him back in shortly. However, when I later called him, he was nowhere to be found. Quickly I put on my coat and searched for him. He had simply vanished.

The next morning I dejectedly arrived at the veterinary hospital. To my surprise I was informed that Bruiser had returned. Curiously enough, he had trudged in the cold winter night for nearly a mile to return to the hospital. A classmate had recognized him at the hospital entrance and brought him in. "Guess he figures that he receives better medical care here," my classmates joked.

"Yeah, he's a traitor," I laughed.

During rounds that morning our advisor mentioned the incident with Bruiser. The instructor was a young pretentious woman. She was a new graduate and eager to gain respect as a faculty member and veterinarian. She was also anxious to display her authority. In front of my classmates she accused me of being irresponsible, especially to let a contagious cat roam freely outdoors. She then said that she didn't want me to take Bruiser back.

My first impulse was to square off with her, toe to toe, face to face. Fortunately I curbed my tongue and informed her that Bruiser wasn't litter trained and that I had merely let him out for a short while so that he could relieve himself. I apologized and stated, "I will not let it reoccur."

"Well, I guess we can let you take him back, but don't let it happen again," she ordered. "I'll give you a second chance."

My undisclosed thought was, "F— you." Instead I offered, "Yes, you're right, and thank you."

Time had arrived to leave WSU and return back to OSU for my final year. Bruiser had finally adjusted to using his litter box and was doing quite well even though he still looked like a veteran prizefighter.

Luckily I had an interim month just to go home and relax. Before leaving I phoned Mom. The mischievous side of me took over. "Mom, I'll be home tomorrow. I'm bringing a dear companion with me. His name is Bruiser — and he has AIDS."

My comment was received with a lengthy silence. Finally Mom muttered, "See you when you get here, drive safely."

When I drove into the driveway, Mom was standing outside waiting. She cautiously scrutinized us. Bruiser was lying next to me on top of the fish tank nonchalantly gazing out the window. Mom carefully stared at us again and then sighed with great relief.

"Thank God it's a cat."

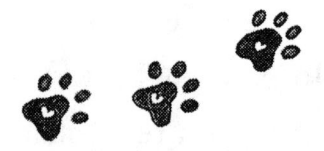

My last year of veterinary school finally arrived. We were required to complete four months of clinical rotations at Oregon State. I completed this task from August through November.

Four students were in my first large animal rotation: Chad Pilgeram, Susan Libra, Brenda Bailey, and myself. Aside from large animal medicine, we set a goal to finish the Portland Marathon race in late September.

We had established the goal earlier that summer. Another classmate, Terri Clark, also trained with us. In fact, she was the instigator for our ambition. Daily we encouraged each other to run until finally the race day arrived.

Completing a marathon is a significant achievement that can only be accomplished one step at a time. In my mind, anyone that participates is a champion, no matter the placement. Finishing was especially important to me. I recalled hardly being able to walk at the end of my freshman year. Now I would finish my experience at OSU by running a marathon. I also thought of my father in a wheelchair and was grateful for the use of my legs and the freedom to run.

All in all the marathon event seemed like an encapsulated version of veterinary school. As long as I kept trying, one step by one step, little by little, enduring to the end, I would eventually finish. And to further enhance the experience, I would be sharing the moment with special friends and classmates.

I realized that with determination, good friends, and endurance, I could most likely achieve whatever I set my mind to. One step at a time.

Sleeping With Angels

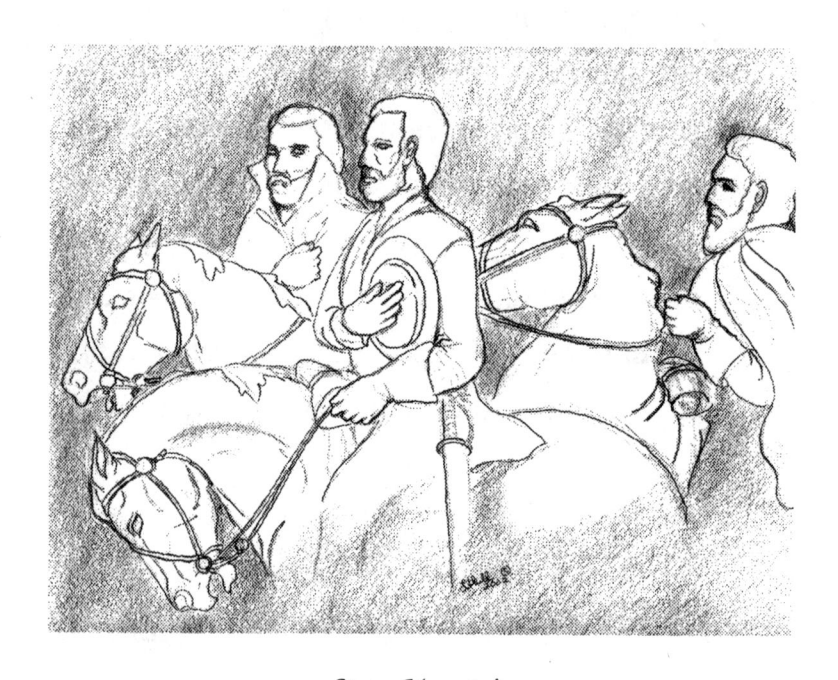

Stone Mountain

5
Freedom

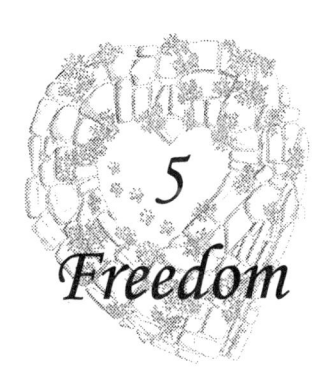

Besides the four months of clinical rotations at OSU, we were also required to complete two months of electives and two months of externships. I completed these requirements from January through April of 1991 at the University of Tennessee School of Veterinary Medicine in Knoxville, Tennessee.

The veterinary school in Tennessee had converted from a three year to four year program. During the transition, in order to effectively staff the teaching hospital, they invited senior veterinary students from around the world to participate in their program. The opportunity was ideal. We were provided expense free living in the dorms, expert teaching staff, and first class teaching facilities. Better still, the juniors were required to perform the nighttime and weekend treatments.

I had driven my 1969 green Ford Custom Fairlane to school. Uncle Jay and Aunt Bareen had sold it to me. The car was like new, in mint condition, and great to travel in. My classmates nicknamed it "the boat" or "the tank." Luckily some of my OSU classmates also participated in the Tennessee program for a few weeks at a time. And we were able to utilize my car to enjoy many weekend road trips together.

On one memorable weekend Tom Timmons, an OSU classmate, and I decided to take a road trip to Atlanta, Georgia. On our way we visited several Civil War sites. We then drove to Stone Mountain State Park outside of Atlanta. On the enormous face of the granite mountain cliffs were carved huge figures of confederate leaders boldly mounted on horses. The breathtaking art piece was magnificent and ghostly.

As we drove out of the park I was still pondering the carvings and their overwhelming presence. The day was quickly descending and the evening twilight brought with it soft rain show-

Freedom

ers. I was driving, filled with thought, and also anxious to reach Atlanta. We hoped to discover what the city looked like while we still had some light. Also we were hungry and wanted to find a good restaurant to have dinner.

I suddenly noticed flashing red lights in my rearview mirror, so I pulled to the side of the road. The patrol car pulled in behind me and a short, overweight police officer approached us. I rolled down my window. Without any introduction he demanded to see my driver's license. His abrupt manner irritated me.

"What's wrong," I challenged.

Again he demanded, without explanation, to see my license.

And again I asked him why he pulled me over.

"Step out of the car immediately," he roared.

Tom glanced at me and suggested that I show the officer my driver's license. I followed his advice and gave my license to the officer.

"Step out of the car now!" he screamed.

"No," I argued, "I gave you my license and you still haven't told me why you pulled me over."

Sleeping With Angels

"I will not tell you again. Step out of your car immediately!"

Again Tom quietly nudged me to obey.

Reluctantly I stepped from the vehicle.

"Stand against the car, face forward with hands placed on the car's hood," he ordered.

"You've got to be kidding," I thought. Turning toward him I again asked why he pulled me over.

As I turned to face him, he immediately reached for his handcuffs and demanded me to face the car with hands behind my back. He then cuffed me and called for backup support. Immediately two other patrol officers arrived.

"Is your friend drunk?" the officer demanded of Tom.

"No, he's a Mormon and doesn't drink alcohol," Tom obediently replied.

The portly officer then readdressed me. "I pulled you over because you were speeding. Now I'm taking you to jail for resisting arrest, threatening an officer, and failure to show your driver's license."

"But I did show..."

"Turn around NOW and shut up," he immediately interrupted.

At that point I realized that I was nothing more than a trapped, angry animal with absolutely no rights.

The officer forced me into the backseat of his car and ordered me to sit on my hands. They soon became uncomfortable and I tried to adjust them. But the slightest movement caused the handcuffs to bite down even tighter on my wrists.

"I'm taking you to DeKalb County Prison in Atlanta," he declared.

I said nothing. I displayed no emotion. I became completely stone cold like the carved figures on the mountain.

Tom followed behind us in the Ford. When we arrived at the county prison the officer escorted me into the secured facilities. After that I no longer saw my friend. Later the guards told me that my buddy had returned to school in Tennessee. They seemed to enjoy relaying the information. I later discovered that Tom had remained all night outside the compound inside my car waiting for my release.

"We're booking you," the officer stated.

After being detained for several hours in a small decaying holding cell, I was mercifully released from confinement. The rotting room contained every type of human discharge imaginable.

My mug shot was then taken. I was stripped and given prison clothes (scrubs) to wear, tested for tuberculosis, and had blood drawn to check for HIV. I was then chained with several other prisoners and marched to another holding cell. In the room were several other men.

Gradually we began to converse with each other. "What are you in here for?" was the common theme.

One black muscular brash teenage man boasted, "A nigger stole my Air Jordan's so I killed him!"

He then glared at me, "What you in for, white boy?"

I meekly replied, "Speeding."

"Speeding! God damn, you're one dumb mother f——, aren't you? How you get yourself put in prison for speeding? Damn!"

The prolonged wait with my questionable fellow prisoners continued into the night. A few cots were in the holding chamber, and some of the inmates slept.

Sleep was the last thing on my mind. Next to staying alive, finding a place to urinate took priority. A couple of toilets were situated openly in the room. I self-consciously relieved myself, flushed the toilet, and observed that the running water was extremely hot. I later discovered the same was true of the showers.

Finally a few of us "less hardened criminals" were ordered to relocate. An older black man had fallen asleep on one of the beds and took a long time to awaken.

"Get up now, nigger!" the uncertain guard yelled as he began to beat the stuporous man.

As the officer raised his arm again to hit the elderly man, I stepped in between him and the prisoner.

"You don't need to do that."

"Let me help you up," I offered to the elderly gentleman.

I was certain that the youthful and impatient prison official would start hitting me. But he sul-

Sleeping With Angels

lenly backed away. To my dismay I soon realized that the older man had defecated and urinated on himself, was drunk, and smelled terrible.

"Give me your left hand," the anxious guard ordered me. "Reach it across your stomach to the right of you and take hold of the stinking nigger's left hand." He then handcuffed us together with my crossed left hand bound to the black man's left hand.

Again I thought of myself as a trapped animal. I soon learned that it was wiser to trust the other prisoners rather than the guards.

Two by two, as handcuffed partners, we were secured to a longer chain that held twelve prisoners. We were transported to different housing areas, which consisted of double wide trailers. These trailers were situated in an immense concrete lot surrounded by high chain link fences crested with razor wire.

Finally unchained, I was escorted to a trailer occupied by thirty-six black men, two Hispanics, and one other Caucasian. I was nervous, to say the least.

I was assigned the top bunk above the other

white prisoner. The metal frame of my bed had no mattress or bedding. "What the hell," I thought, "I'm certainly not going to sleep anyway."

"What you in here for, white boy?" They laughed when I told them. From what I could safely determine, most of the men were charged with misdemeanors or less serious crimes, such as delinquent child support, driving under the influence, and oh yes, speeding. No murderers, sexual deviants, or psychopaths as far as I could determine.

Even so, I knew I did not feel safe going to sleep.

The building contained a phone, television, and restroom with only scalding hot water. Interestingly enough, toilet paper was nowhere to be found. I learned that the inmates valued it as a premium and hid the rolls like treasure underneath their mattresses. Thankfully I didn't need to use any.

Fortunately we were allowed one phone call so I hurriedly phoned home. Mom answered on the second ring.

"Will you accept charges from Alan Cunningham?" the operator asked.

Sleeping With Angels

"Yes, yes," Mom impatiently stated. "How's school?" she asked. "It's so good to hear from you. You're always in our prayers."

"Mom," I confided, "I'm in prison in Atlanta, Georgia." The resulting silence seemed an eternity.

Eventually she gasped. "You're where? Oh, my god! What are you doing in prison?"

"Mom, I only have a minute. Can you phone Jim; he has a lawyer friend that might be able to help me."

Silence.

"Mom, are you there?"

I heard her in the background yelling to Dad, "Alan's in prison. Get Jimmy right now!"

She had simply dropped the phone and forgotten to hang it up.

Finally an officer brought me a mattress, pillow, and bedding. I barely leaned back on my bed when several guards entered the building. At three a.m. they were taking us to breakfast! We were shackled to a lengthy chain and marched to the dining room area. The main course was grits. Afterwards, we were then escorted, with restraints, back to the trailer.

Freedom

Later that morning, while most of the men were sleeping, others were watching basketball on television. I decided to watch. Some of the men asked what I was doing in Georgia. I told them that I was mainly in the area to finish veterinary school. They seemed to nod their heads with new respect towards me.

Slowly, one by one, the other inmates retired to bed or morning showers. Since I was the lone television audience or so I thought, I began to channel surf. When I noted a figure skating program, I happily established myself to enjoy the remainder of the event. I love watching this artistic sport.

Now I think back and realize that changing the television program from basketball to figure skating was nothing short of a death wish. I can only guess that the other "hardened criminals" must have thought I was either crazy or possessed balls of steel. No one challenged my choice of programs.

"Alan Cunningham," a voice faintly echoed. I was so engrossed with the television that I didn't realize I was being summoned. "Please follow me,"

Sleeping With Angels

the guard interrupted. Quickly I came to my senses and jumped up. He then led me, unshackled, to the judge.

Miraculously, my brother Jim had communicated with his attorney friend, Gerald Conder. Likewise, my friend Tom had phoned my brother Bob, who was living in New Orleans at the time with his family. We had previously stayed with them on a weekend Mardi Gras celebration. Due to their combined efforts they were able to obtain my prison release.

Before I was liberated, I was again kept in a holding cell with several other inmates where we were given our personal belongings. Interestingly enough, while waiting for discharge, the majority of the inmates were planning their next crime.

I had endured nearly twenty-four hours in prison confinement. The experience is one I'll never forget. I learned nothing more than to further resent supposed "authority figures" who wield power with little accountability. I felt violated by their system. And although the incarceration period was a relatively short amount of time, what I felt and experienced will forever remain.

While leaving the compound with Tom, who had been patiently waiting for me from the beginning of the entire ordeal, one of the other liberated inmates approached me.

"Hey Al, can I have a couple of bucks for a bus ticket?"

"Sure," I acknowledged and offered him bus fare.

"So they know you on a first name basis," Tom jokingly observed.

"Yes," I laughed nervously and then felt something new.

The sense of freedom, which I normally took for granted, was overpowering.

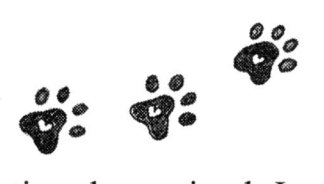

At last, graduation day arrived. I crossed the finish line and accomplished my goal with the help of many wonderful people. And even though the goal took longer than normal, I completed it one step at a time.

I was notoriously and respectfully branded by my classmates as the bald headed, old man, ex con

Mormon, to which I proudly replied, "Don't mess with me, I now have low friends in low places."

"I suppose it will take an all points bulletin to communicate with you," one fellow student good-naturedly mocked.

"Just don't call collect," I returned.

Nearing completion of the graduation ceremony, with diploma in hand, we recited the veterinary oath together.

"Being admitted to the profession of veterinary medicine,

I solemnly swear to use my scientific knowledge and skills for the benefit of society through the protection of animal health, the relief of animal suffering, the conservation of livestock resources, the promotion of public health, and the advancement of medical knowledge.

I will practice my profession conscientiously, with dignity, and in keeping with the principles of veterinary medical ethics.

I accept as a lifelong obligation the continual improvement of my professional knowledge and competence."

Adapted by the American Veterinary Medical Association House of Delegates, July 1969.

How did I feel? Silently I concluded that armed with a diploma and an extensive formal education to guide me, I now had the freedom to choose my future as a veterinarian. But to my amazement, after graduation I discovered I was burned out and empty of any desire to practice.

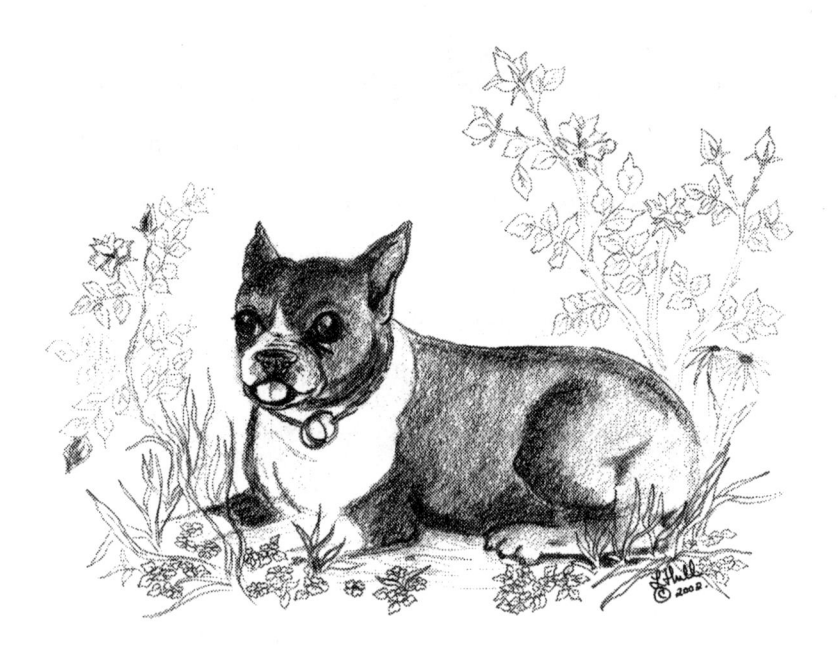

Pug

6
Pug

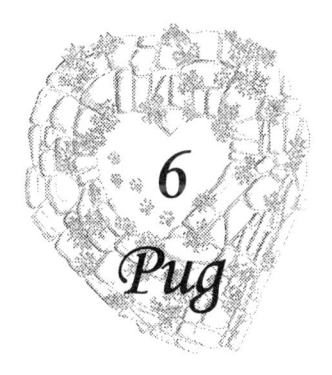

Thankfully I had graduated from veterinary school and was now home for good. "No more school forever," I celebrated. I was free from exams, assignments, and deadlines — or so I thought. I was thirty-five years old, single, grossly in debt, living with my parents, overeducated, and unemployed. In short, I was nothing more than a detriment to society.

Sarcasm aside, although I deeply missed the companionship of my classmates, I was happy to be home. Essentially, I was burned out from school. Sometimes it's good to step away from yourself long enough to take inventory and to appreciate what you really have. I had my health, family, friends, and my animals. Basically I considered my animals to be my family since I was single.

Truly I possessed the greatest treasures of life!

Since Dad and Mom had so graciously supported me through the long haul of school, I felt that it was now my turn to help them. Dad was getting weaker. Mom required help transferring him in his wheelchair. Also Dad's speech was becoming slurred and more difficult to understand.

Furthermore, besides directly helping my parents, I also enjoyed jogging, traveling, gardening, oil painting, maintaining the house, and being with my animals. All in all, the refreshing activities away from school seemed to rejuvenate and revitalize me. And I actually began to entertain the thought of practicing veterinary medicine.

As far as my precious animals were concerned, One Step was still greeting us with his cheerful songs. Besides singing, I also discovered that he loved to be held and fed soda crackers.

Bruiser had taken up residence on the side porch. Because of his feline aids virus, he constantly had an upper respiratory infection even though I continually treated him. But he never complained and remained my trooper.

Some of my other animals such as China Doll,

Tapioca, and Licorice had died several years prior. Other now gone beloved animals included two dogs, Blackie and Yort, and a crippled cat named Mama.

Moreover, while I was enrolled in veterinary school I had three dogs at home. Dad and Mom had taken superb care of them while I was gone. Their names were Alamosa, Ginger, and Jaws. Part way through school at Washington State, Alamosa died from old age. Alamosa, as always, had remained intrigued with flying objects. Shortly following, Ginger died with heart failure.

But I still had Jaws. She was a cross between a Weimaraner and Doberman Pinscher. The year previous she had an aggressive mast cell tumor removed from her back. Chest radiographs revealed some questionable lung nodules. I sadly doubted how much quality of life Jaws had remaining. But for the time being, she appeared happy and eager to be with me, and I with her.

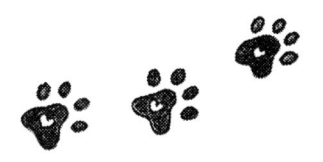

Shortly after returning home I began to work at a

long-term health care center Doxey Hatch, as a respiratory therapist. Some of the chronic patients were trached and maintained on mechanical ventilators due to closed head injury, near drowning, or end stage chronic obstructive pulmonary disease.

By this time my desire to practice veterinary medicine was rekindled and I hoped to practice soon. But I still needed to pass my national boards. The exams weren't offered until December, which was six months away. And as luck would have it, the closest facility to take the exams was at Colorado State University. I boldly determined that during my free time at Doxey Hatch, I would diligently study for the national boards and prepare to successfully pass them.

Looking back, I vividly recall a lengthy hallway in Doxey Hatch. Housed at the end of the mysterious and dark corridor were several patients dying of AIDS. Seldom did I see any of them outside of their rooms. Occasionally I would be called by the nurses to suction the secretions from the airways of those who suffered from pneumonia.

Curiously, after some time, I wanted to know more about the people hidden within the lonely rooms. I quietly walked to the end of the dark hall and peered into the quarters. Amazed, I soon discovered that the patients afflicted with AIDS had very different presentations of this fatal disease.

The deathly face of AIDS, for example, was frightfully expressed as black and furry candida fungal colonies covering the body, reptile-like skin lesions, pneumocystis carini pneumonia, dementia, and skin cancer, just to list a few.

Sadly enough, I also discovered that as grotesque as the terminal affects of HIV were presented, the most heartbreaking effect of the disease was the ostracization that the patients were forced to endure. Many were abandoned by their family, spouse, lover, or others. They faced the challenge of death alone.

"No one should have to face death alone," I reasoned. Unfortunately, even today, some people choose to fight the carriers of the disease rather than the disease itself.

When I had the opportunity, I would visit with the patients that were healthy enough to have company, and just listen to them, or simply share their photographs of happier times. Frequently we would leisurely proceed outside to sit in the sun, or to drink a soda pop. Periodically, a few patients would ask me to accompany them to an area where they could smoke a cigarette.

I greatly valued the time shared with them, and learned to respect the AIDS patients for the admirable way many of them courageously confronted impending death.

Today, due to improved drugs and medical regimens, more HIV patients are surviving. Through gaining more knowledge, and learning to battle the disease rather than the carriers, I hope that someday we can completely destroy the monstrous face of AIDS — here and around the world.

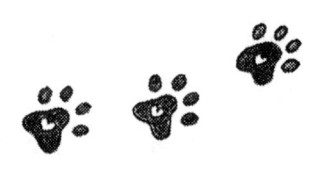

Late December and national board exams both arrived all too soon. I was determined to travel to Colorado State University, take the veterinary exams, and return home successful. Only this time I would take a lucky charm — Jaws, my loyal friend and canine companion.

Steadfastly she remained by my side and was

my constant support. Across the cold, windblown Wyoming plains we journeyed and arrived in Ft. Collins the next day. Each night Jaws cuddled next to me. Her comforting warmth gave me fortitude to face my tests with positive determination. I was certain that with an angel by my side, I could only succeed.

Following two days of exhausting exams we returned home. I felt relieved and confident. In February I received my passing scores. As is so common with life, bitter and sweet are often intertwined — Jaws died a few days after I learned I had passed the national boards.

Jaws had faithfully endured with me to the end. I had obtained her just before I started veterinary school at Colorado State and she freely offered me a lifetime of her strength and support.

When she knew that I was able to stand alone, she quietly said goodbye. To make sure that I was okay, however, she soon sent me another guardian angel. Her name was Pug.

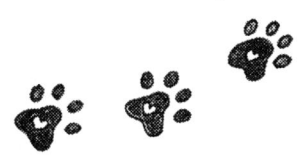

Sleeping With Angels

On my parents living room bookshelf rested a photograph of Dad and Mom when they were first married. Dad was holding a small, black and white pug-nosed dog.

"That's Mitzie," Dad informed as he pointed to the dog. "I had her when me and your mom got married. She used to sit on the back of my car seat next to my shoulder when I was driving. Often, as she sat perched next to me, she would let farts and then playfully spin in circles chasing her stubby tail," he laughed. "Me and your mom got the biggest kick out of her."

"What breed of dog was she?" I asked.

"Just a pug dog."

After carefully examining her picture I corrected, "I think she's a Boston Terrier."

"Whatever" Dad replied, "I sure loved that pug dog."

Dad reminisced to me about Mitzie several times as I was growing up. Now I was older, finished with veterinary school, and I wanted to try and repay my parents for their long suffering support.

As I observed Dad in his wheelchair, he

seemed very sad and lonely. After all, he had worked for several years on his walking route as a postal carrier. "He must be very frustrated to not have the use of his legs," I reflected.

"Dad, would you like another dog like Mitzie?" I asked.

His eyes brightened! "Oh boy, would I," he struggled in his slurred speech.

"Then I will find you one." I thought a Boston Terrier would make a wonderful companion and lap dog for dad. Little did I appreciate how much energy they possessed.

Mom overheard me and quietly warned, "I think we better give it some time."

To no avail. Dad and I, both stubborn Scotsmen, had made up our minds. And Mom quickly realized that she was wasting her time in trying to change us.

I was also thinking of myself. Jaws was gone and I was unhappy without a dog. I craved the companionship of another.

The next day I drove to Hailstone Pet Store in Provo. A friend had informed me that they might have Boston Terriers. When I arrived I mentioned to the store manager what I was searching for. She enthusiastically replied, "Follow me, I have just what you want!"

Excited, I followed. In a glass enclosure were several Boston Terrier puppies. One was slightly bigger and older than the others. She caught my attention immediately. Her beautiful black, almond-shaped eyes beckoned with curiosity and mischievousness. In my heart I felt that Jaws had carefully selected the best dog angel from heaven and sent her to me to be my new companion.

"The larger pup is the last of her litter; I would like to find a good home for her if you're interested."

I announced to the clerk that I was sold on the larger pup long before she said anything.

"Wonderful. I'm sure that you will like her. Let me give you her pedigree chart."

I noted that she was born August 21, 1991, to Casey's Little Mike (sire), and Tooter's Lil Chubby (dam). The breeder's name was Donald Peay from American Fork, Utah.

"How interesting," I thought, "My home town."

"If you'd like, you can mail in these papers, along with the fee, to have her registered."

Honestly, I just wanted another companion. Papers, pedigrees, and registrations weren't important.

Tenderly I carried my new little girl out to the car. She timidly curled up on my lap for the ride home. When we arrived I presented her to Dad. "Here's your baby. What are you going to name her?" I asked.

With a broad smile he clearly announced, "Pug."

"But she's a Boston Terrier. Don't you think we should name her something different?"

Even though he was in a wheelchair, Dad would not be ordered. Again he clearly stated, "Pug."

"Then Pug is her name," I agreed.

"Oh, Jim," Mom argued, "can't you think of something more dainty, she's a little girl." Easily we could see that mom had fallen in love with her as much as we had.

"No, her name is Pug," Dad sternly repeated.

"I guess we'll call her Pug then," Mom sighed.

At first she seemed shy and overwhelmed by her new environment. I placed her on Dad's lap. She just lay there with her large eyes taking in the surroundings. Dad held her gently, rubbing her head. For the first time in a long while he had a contented look on his face.

Technically I had given Pug to dad. But in my heart, she belonged to me. She had tugged on my heartstrings from the moment I saw her. The shiny black and white markings, the short fur, the spherical belly, the narrow white stripe running from her stubby nose to her forehead, the rounded posterior without a tail, the broken little toe on her left front foot, the broad shoulders, the naturally cropped ears, the tiny accent of pink tongue protruding from her mouth, the slightest under bite, and most of all the exquisitely bright and beautiful enormous black eyes. In my mind I memorized every inch of my newest friend and companion.

That night Pug crawled into bed with me. Inquisitively she tunneled under the covers and then snuggled closer and closer against my stomach.

"Are you comfortable, little girl?" I asked while patting her tiny round head. She replied by warmly licking my hand. Never before had I felt so safe, peaceful, and relaxed. For I had a precious gift next to me. I was sleeping with an angel.

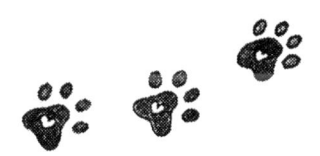

Now that I had officially passed my national boards I could begin work as a veterinarian and also prepare to take state boards. I was both excited and apprehensive to begin practice. With renewed determination I looked forward to starting my profession and actively realizing my lifetime dream. In addition, possibly as a sense of security, I continued to work as a respiratory therapist.

Stepping into the real world of veterinary medicine was an arena totally different from school. At times I doubted if my formal education had effectively prepared me for the real thing.

The state licensing division required new veterinarians to work as interns with a licensed veterinarian for six months or one thousand hours.

The owner and veterinarian of the first hospital where I worked, catered to dog breeders and show dog owners. What an impossible audience for a new graduate to please. "If this is what veterinary medicine is all about, I want nothing to do with it," I announced to myself.

I soon found that I worked more than forty hours a week at the veterinary clinic, in addition to thirty-six hours every weekend as a respiratory therapist.

One day the owner of the veterinary clinic bargained, "I need you here more. You must choose between veterinary medicine and respiratory care."

I easily selected respiratory care, and somehow felt that he knew the same before even asking me to make the decision. After four and one half months, I left my first veterinary job.

Since I had successfully completed the state boards a few weeks prior to my termination, I approached the state licensing committee about becoming licensed. They indicated that the policy specifically stated that six months or one thousand hours be completed by the intern before receiving a state license. I argued that I might not have completed six months but I certainly had worked one thousand hours.

I reminded them that the rules indicated six

months or one thousand hours, not six months and one thousand hours. But they refused to listen and firmly stated that I must complete one thousand hours of work within a six-month period — no more, no less. I stated that the rules needed to be more specifically and accurately worded. Instead of reasoning with me, they became irritated by my challenge and refused to discuss it any further. I left the meeting and my profession with a rekindled distrust for some of the people in veterinary medicine and authority figures who seemingly misused their power.

Some two years later I returned again to veterinary medicine and worked at the Utah Humane Society. The experience provided many chances to perform vaccinations and spay or neuter surgeries. But my heart broke when I saw the hopeful and eager eyes of all the homeless animals.

And sadly, I realized the majority of them would not find a home. The true fact of the matter was that nearly seventy percent of the sheltered animals would be euthanized. Seeing this day in and day out, I vowed to encourage pet sterilization.

The policy of the humane society was somewhat different to my perception of quality veterinary medicine. According to the manager's conservative and practical money-saving custom, she would rather euthanize a sick animal than medically treat it. In my eager and optimistic style I would rather treat and give the animal a chance. I suppose that neither of us were completely wrong or right; it's just that both of us were too stubborn to compromise. In the end, I left the humane society after working there four and one half months.

As a veterinarian I am grateful that euthanasia is available for terminally pain-filled and sick animals. I also wish that human medicine would offer the same mercy to hopelessly ill patients. It seems inconceivable to me that as a society, we recognize the kindness of putting a suffering animal out of its misery, yet we are completely willing for a human being to suffer endlessly.

Dog's Prayer
by Beth Norman Harris

Treat me kindly, my beloved master, for no heart in all the world is more grateful for kindness than the loving heart of me.

Do not break my spirit with a stick, for though I should lick your hand between the blows, your patience and understanding will more quickly teach me the things you would have me to do.

Speak to me often, for your voice is the world's sweetest music, as you must know by the fierce wagging of my tail when your footstep falls upon my waiting ear.

When it is cold and wet, please take me inside, for I am now a domesticated animal, no longer used to bitter elements. And I ask no greater glory than the privilege of sitting at your feet beside the hearth. Though had you no home,

I would rather follow you through ice and snow than rest upon the softest pillow in the warmest home in all the land, for you are my god, and I your devoted worshiper. Keep my pan filled with fresh water, for although I should not reproach you were it dry, I cannot tell you when I suffer thirst. Feed me clean food, that I may stay well, to romp and play and do your bidding, to walk by your side and stand ready, willing and able to protect you with my life should your life be in danger.

And, beloved master, should the great Master see fit to deprive me of my health or sight, do not turn me away from you. Rather hold me gently in Your arms as skilled hands grant me the merciful boon of eternal rest – and I will leave you knowing with the last breath I drew, my fate was ever safest in your hands.

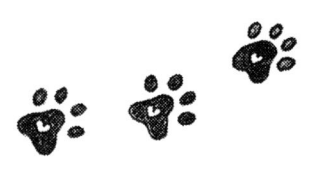

Nearly four years had transpired since graduating from Oregon State Veterinary College, and I was still striving to obtain my state license. According to the licensing authorities I was six weeks shy of the required six months of internship necessary to receive a license.

Again I interviewed with the licensing committee. They politely introduced themselves along with their attorney.

I again argued that I should be allowed a Utah State veterinary license: "Between the two veterinary positions, I have completed over six months and one thousand hours of internships."

The committee chairman, who was not a veterinarian (most of the other members were) stated, "According to the guidelines you must complete the six months and one thousand hours within a one year period."

I replied, "I have not seen that policy in the rules and regulations."

"Perhaps you can discuss this with our attorney," the chairman smugly stated.

The attorney promptly explained the new and amended laws. "We will allow you three months to complete the remaining six weeks," he offered.

As the committee members were discussing my options a gentleman messenger knocked on the door to the room, "Please excuse me," he apologized, "but I have an urgent message for the committee chairman."

Abruptly the chairman requested, "What is it?"

"Could I deliver the information to you privately," the messenger meekly suggested.

Sharply the chairman yelled, "Just tell me what you want, now!"

Embarrassed, the messenger stated, "I need to inform you that you are running late for your next meeting. I'm so sorry for the intrusion."

Impatiently the chairman brushed the intruder aside and turned to me. "Do you think that you should be paid for working as a veterinary intern and if so why?"

"Yes," I warily replied. "I am providing a professional service to the pub…"

"What do you think about it, Mr. Attorney," he rudely interrupted.

"No. Accord…"

"Wait one moment," I intervened. "You did not allow me an opportunity to complete my answer."

"You just wait now," the chairman angrily countered.

"No!" I had lost control. "You are an extremely rude person. And as far as I'm concerned, you can go to hell!"

Immediately the chairman catapulted from his chair. Slamming his notebook on the table, he exclaimed, "This is a waste of my time!" Enraged he stomped out of the room.

I watchfully sat in silence.

"Do you know who that was," the committee secretary charged. "He is the final person to okay your license. I am going to red flag your file immediately. In fact, I will see to it that you can't obtain a veterinary license anywhere in the country."

"Bullshit!" I silently boiled.

The kangaroo court had begun. One by one, each remaining member harassed me with unnec-

Sleeping With Angels

essary and cheap verbal shots. Silently I listened, unable to believe what was happening.

Ultimately, one committee member announced, "I think this meeting is over. We will get back with you."

"Fine," I conceded, then defiantly slammed the door behind me as I marched out. I angrily proceeded to my car outside, then shamefully wondered, "What just happened? What an unprofessional experience."

Mercifully Pug was waiting in the car for me. She had become my constant companion. "You know, little girl," I stubbornly realized, "I have a problem of saying the wrong thing to the wrong person at the wrong time. I resent authority figures. I refuse to automatically respect anyone until they earn it. I would much rather fight for the underdog."

Soon tears streamed from my eyes. Peacefully a warm, gentle touch quietened me. "You will be okay buddy, don't worry," Pug seemed to comfort as she licked the tears from my face.

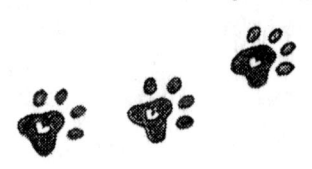

Fortunately, the licensing committee kept true to their word and allowed me three more months to complete six weeks or two hundred and forty hours of internship. Dr. Cliff Ziegenhorn, a nighttime emergency veterinarian in Salt Lake City, allowed me to complete my hours with him. Nearly thirteen years after I first entered veterinary school, I finally received my license.

What a challenging endeavor. Again I reflected if it was worth the turmoil. If it meant anything towards having Pug, without hesitation I would have to say a resounding "Yes."

Sleeping With Angels

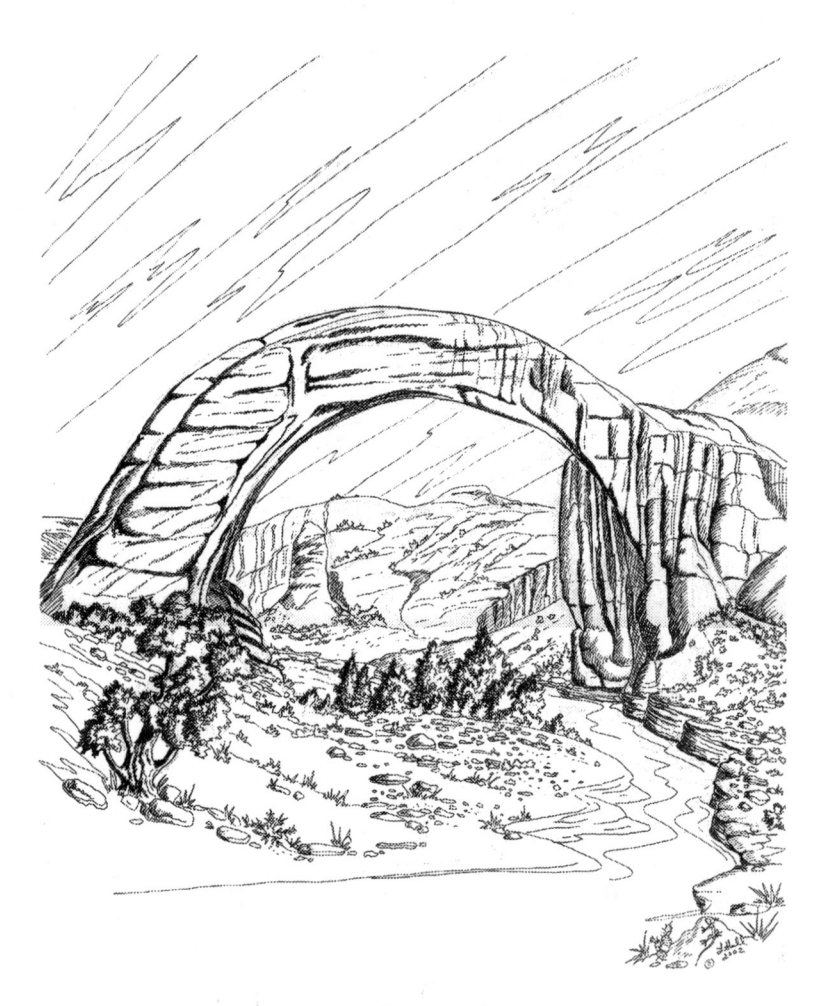

Rainbow Bridge

7
Small Wonders

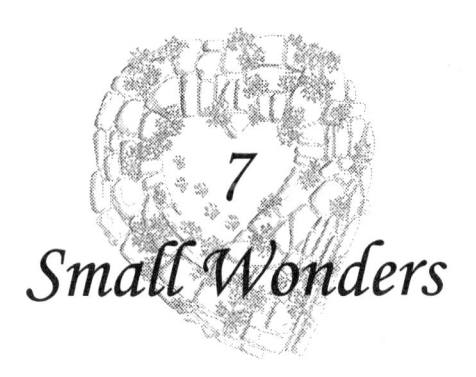

"We are all travelers in the wilderness of the world, and the best we find in our travels is an honest friend." Robert Louis Stevenson

Besides working as a veterinarian, I also maintained another lifetime goal: to see the natural and manmade wonders of the world. Fortunately, after graduating from Oregon State University, I was able to pursue that goal. Quite frankly, if I had to compare, I would value the education gained from travel more than the education received from formal schooling. Not only that, the traveling experiences were much more enjoyable, interesting, and relaxing. And oh yes, also much less expensive. Two wonders that I especially recollect are Rainbow Bridge, in Utah, and Taj Mahal, in India.

Rainbow Bridge (Nonnezoshe), nestled in the protective shadows of Navajo Mountain near the Utah and Arizona border, is the world's largest natural stone bridge. The sandstone arch is two hundred and ninety feet tall with a two hundred and seventy-five foot long span. This is large enough to comfortably fit the entire United States Capitol Building underneath.

The Navajo Indians consider the multi-hued sandstone arch to be sacred. Legend holds that Nonnezoshe (rainbow turned to stone) was created when an inchworm caterpillar (shooting worm) stretched itself across the canyon. The resulting span provided a bridge to the Navajo Twin Gods.

Many traditional American Indians have superstitious beliefs about the natural archway. To some it is the sign of the sun's course over the earth. Others consider the Rainbow Bridge to be the doorway between life and death. Still others believe that it is forbidden to walk underneath the sacred arch without saying a special prayer.

Since the land between Navajo Mountain and Rainbow Bridge is also considered sacred, the national park service has officially eliminated all maps and pamphlets that explain how to hike to the monument. Presently the rugged trails into the stone arch are still open to the public, but are extremely difficult to maneuver.

"One can easily get lost in the vast canyons leading to Rainbow Bridge," wrote Zane Grey. The great western novelist described his journey in 1913 as one of the worst trails in the West. He recorded the land to be a "chaos of a million canyons, where a man became nothing."

In late September 1995, my friend Rob and I challenged ourselves to hike the sixteen miles into the desolate canyons of Navajo Nation. Being somewhat adventurous, stubborn, and foolhardy (simply put — men,) we chose to traverse the poorly marked, rugged trails leading into the sacred structure, rather than to procure a simpler tourist boat ride on Lake Powell into the natural wonder.

We enthusiastically started our journey early in the morning. The expansive blue sky was crisp and clear. Armed with hiking gear we looked forward to experiencing the pristine scenery. The massive, sheer canyon cliffs were vibrant with brilliant sandstone orange, red, yellow, black, and vermilion. The barren landscape of red sand was accented with sagebrush, cedars, volcanic rock, and a few cottonwood trees near the occasional streams. Some of the leaves had already turned a stunning amber.

Of course, my constant companion, Pug, accompanied us. Initially she was aglow with puppy enthusiasm as she explored the new surroundings, smiling and running up and down the obscure trails. Eventually, however, she tired. Convincingly she situated herself in front of me and pleadingly looked up.

"Okay little girl, I'll carry you," I resigned.

Pug beamed as she was now able to get a better view of the scenery without expending the least bit of energy. Sometimes I would try to cradle her next to my shoulder. But she wouldn't allow it. She must face forward in order to see what waited ahead.

Therefore she rested, her front legs draped across my outstretched left arm, and her hindquarters nestled on my right arm. When I became tired she would briefly tolerate walking and then would again move in front of me, stop, and beg to be carried. Again, I picked her up and carried her.

Onward we steadfastly marched. The mid-day sun became uncomfortably hot. Eventually we arrived at the top of a narrow, rocky trail tightly clinging to the side of the steep cliffs. Pug and I cautiously continued the weaving descent downwards, but Rob would not move.

"What's wrong," I yelled back.

"I can't do it," Rob replied.

"Do what?" I asked.

"I'm afraid of heights," he admitted.

The mischievous smirk on my face soon disappeared. Returning back to Rob I offered to let him hold onto my arm so that we could descend the perilous canyon path together.

"No, you and Pug go on. I'll meet you back at the campsite where the truck is."

Warily I agreed. "Pug and I will continue on then." Silently we watched as the physical giant of a man slowly turned around and left us.

Sleeping With Angels

Early afternoon beckoned and we still hadn't reached Rainbow Bridge. "Just a little ways further," I encouraged. Pug just looked up at me with complete confidence.

"Besides, as long as you carry me, I'm with you all the way buddy," her eyes seemed to convey.

Finally we discovered a small canyon with running water. We drank and rested. I noted the afternoon shade was stretching across the canyon. "The sun is starting to descend, Pug, I think we better turn around."

Disappointed, we turned back. On another future occasion Pug and I were able to successfully reach Rainbow Bridge. This time, however, we didn't. After filling our water container in the refreshing stream we started our lone, arduous journey back.

My goal was to ascend out of the deep canyon my friend had left us at before nightfall. I decided that particular area of the hike would be much too treacherous to navigate in the dark. Fortunately we climbed out of the canyon as dusk approached. The remaining trail back to camp was fairly flat and more easily passable.

The vast skies gradually continued to darken and storm clouds gathered. Then it began to rain. Unfortunately, I had no flashlight. The poorly marked trails became impossible to follow in the dark.

"Pug, I need your help to find our way back. I'm lost and can't see very well. You're going to have to walk ahead and guide us to camp."

Exhausted, I placed her on the ground. She looked up at me as if to say, "We can do it buddy." She shook the rain off herself, and then confidently marched ahead, one step at a time. I followed with complete trust in her. Frequently she would stop, look back at me to see that I was okay, and then proceed forward.

After several hours in the darkened, rainy evening we arrived to the path that led to our campsite and truck. Not once, during that entire time, did Pug beg me to carry her. And when she safely guided us to the roughened dirt road she then began to walk faster. "We made it buddy," she seemed to rejoice, "I'm so excited to be back!"

"Pug, you are my little wonder," I proudly acknowledged to her.

Sleeping With Angels

Rob greeted us at the truck. He had prepared dinner. "I was worried if you would make it back in the dark."

I told him about Pug being our guide.

He grinned, "She is some dog."

"Yes," I agreed. Truly she had been my guiding light and faithful companion. I also realized that without Pug, alone in the merciless canyons, I would have become "nothing."

After we ate I gently placed Pug on the front seat of the truck. She quickly fell asleep, and soon afterwards I did as well. We peacefully slept next to each other as Rob drove us back home to the comforts of modern civilization.

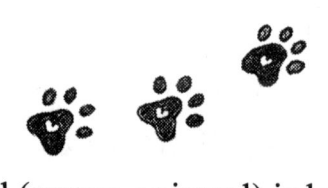

The Taj Mahal (crown or jewel) is located in Agra, India, about one hundred miles southeast of the national capital New Delhi. Although the distance from New Delhi to Agra is relatively short, the journey by road is an all day affair.

The main connecting road is constantly under construction and repair due to the damage caused from the yearly monsoons. Along the route is a dichotomous mixture of old and new: heavy road machinery, men working with shovels and wheelbarrows, camel drawn carts, cattle, bicycles, small cars, and brilliantly clothed Indians.

I eventually arrived in Agra. The wondrous Taj Mahal can not only be appreciated from a distance, it can also be admired close up in detail.

Emperor Shah Jahan had the white marble edifice, or tomb, constructed in memory of his beloved wife, Mumtaz Mahal, in 1629. He employed 20,000 workers from India, Asia, and Europe to create the Taj Mahal. Completion time required twenty-two years.

The gem like beauty of the Taj Mahal is considered by many as the most beautiful and perfectly built building in the world. The delicately sculpted marble walls are etched with elaborate floral designs that are adorned with semiprecious stones such as agates, jasper, bloodstones, and coral. Needless to say, the painstaking detail is remarkably exquisite.

During my visit to the magnificent shrine, I stayed nearby at the Taj Mahal Hotel. This was a luxurious, modern building with mostly Caucasian or upper class Indian guests.

My personal tour guide Hassan, who was a native Indian, accompanied me to the hotel. I invited him to stay with me and he seemed to respond favorably. While I was checking in, Hassan waited for me outside. After making arrangements with the clerk for an extra person, I proceeded out to obtain my luggage and to invite my tour guide into the lodging with me.

As I approached the hotel's entrance I witnessed a troubling event. The doorman and several of the facility managers were hitting my friend with their fists. Hassan was crying in fear and pain. Immediately I charged onto the steps and ordered the men to leave him alone. "He is my guest!" I shouted.

"But he's a commoner," they quickly returned. "We have luggage waiting next to the hotel entrance and we are suspicious that he will steal something."

"No, he won't," I retaliated. I was ready to demand my money back and to stay somewhere else. But before my threat was released, Hassan tearfully glanced at me and offered, "I have friends close by that I can stay with, I'll be okay, don't worry. I will see you tomorrow around nine a.m."

I sadly realized that I could not change several hundred years of caste tradition. I didn't like what I thought was extremely unfair, but realistically I could do nothing about it. Perhaps the same type of exclusive judgment exists in America, only not as obvious.

The next morning, Hassan was waiting for me in the hotel parking lot, patiently standing next to his compact car. With a broad smile he approached, took me by the hand, and accompanied me back to his vehicle.

I awkwardly apologized again for the events of the day before. "No problem," he reminded me. "We will have a good day," he assured.

Reflecting back, I realized the wondrous communicating power of his small and simple gesture of holding my hand. And it seemed to me that the great tragedy of our society is that men are taught to clench a fist before they open a hand. How unfortunate that it is more acceptable to see men hit each other then to hold hands.

Sleeping With Angels

I have often imagined what life would be like without caste systems, malice, phobias, governments, religions, wealth, and poverty. John Lennon's immensely popular and universal song "Imagine" exemplifies my feelings.

> *"You may say I'm a dreamer*
> *But I'm not the only one*
> *I hope someday you'll join us*
> *And the world will be as one."*

From the song, "Imagine" by John Lennon

Sleeping With Angels

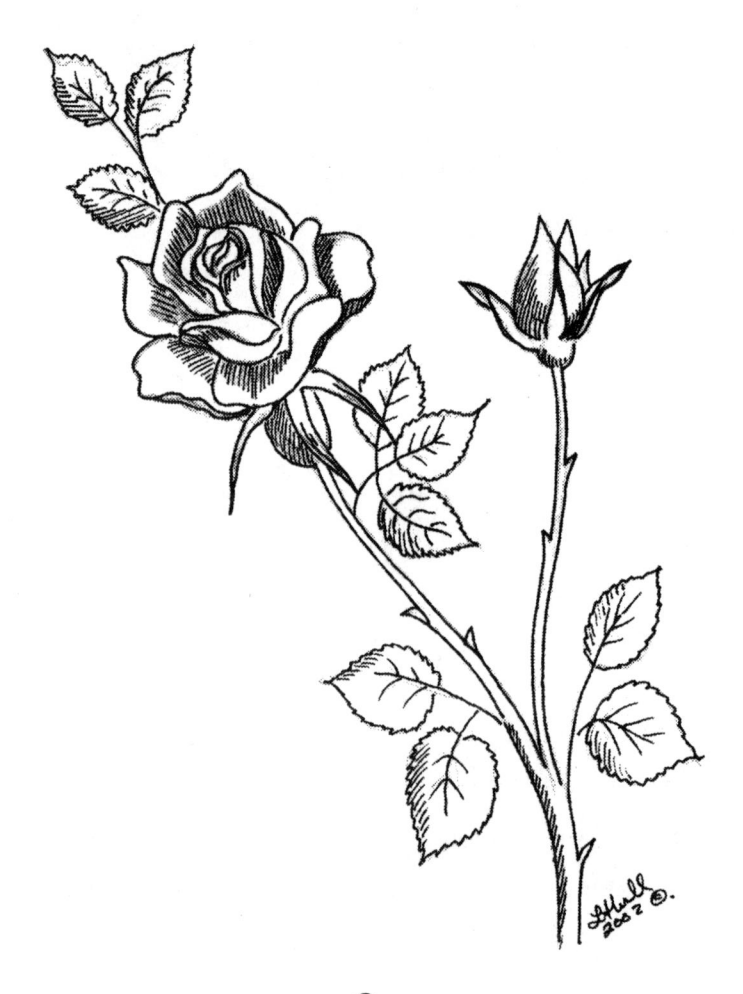

Rose

8
Farewell

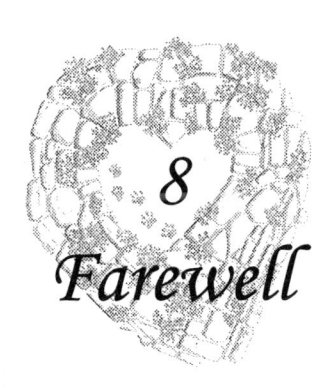

One Step had faithfully greeted us with his joyous morning salutations for nearly fifteen years. And we counted on hearing it.

None of us could ever forget One Step's rugged beginnings. "What can a bird do without a leg and wing," I had said when I discovered the tiny bird struggling in the cold water. As I felt his suffering, I thought it would be best to destroy him.

"Don't, Uncle! He acts like he wants to live," Jan gasped.

And live he did! One Step's courageous lifespan extended nearly three years beyond the normal for cockatiels. His bright and cheerful demeanor brought inspiration and happiness to many people. The example of his wholehearted determination had given me resolution when I was

Sleeping With Angels

weak. Too often, with my busy work schedule as a relief veterinarian and respiratory therapist, I regretfully didn't pay enough attention to him.

Strangely, my active conscience sometimes ignored his beautiful music and jovial announcements. Interestingly enough, when he was noisy I didn't hear him, but when he was quiet I listened.

This particular morning when I awoke, I didn't hear his usual greetings. There was only silence. "What's wrong with One Step?" I wondered. "He's so unusually quiet." I arose from bed to check on him and found him lying dead on the floor of his cage. "One Step," I groaned. "You seemed okay last night." And I deeply regretted that I could no longer listen to his cheerful salutations.

Carefully I wrapped him in a handkerchief and silently buried him in the pet cemetery with my other former beloved pet companions. The burial grounds were located behind my parents' house near the rose gardens. Mom and my nephew Troy had tenderly constructed a solitary headstone for the cemetery when Alamosa died. They created a beautiful monument from sandstone and quartz rocks.

Mom watched as I buried One Step. She quietly informed me that she noticed he had passed away earlier that morning, but she didn't want to awaken me. Mom had appropriately given One Step his name. She would often deny it, but she eventually became attached to all of my animals. I knew she was as upset about his death as I was.

With the joy of being blessed with loving companions comes the heartache of losing them. One Step had changed my life. I would never forget him.

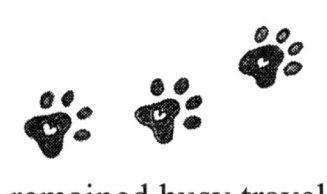

Commonly, I remained busy traveling the state of Utah as a relief veterinarian. After obtaining my state license I was allowed to work alone. Frequently, Dr. David Pearson, at Roy Veterinary Hospital, asked me to cover for him when he was gone. He trusted me and that meant a lot.

I determined that working as a relief veterinarian was the best way to go for me. I was able to work where I liked — and when I wanted. I managed to stay too busy and had to learn to say "no" sometimes. I continued working weekend nights as a respiratory therapist.

One late afternoon I arrived home worn out as usual. Mom quickly informed me that Bruiser was sick and lying on my bed. She said the neighbor had discovered him semiconscious on her front porch and had contacted her. Mom wrapped Bruiser in a towel and carried him home.

Earlier that week I had noticed Bruiser wasn't eating much. And that troubled me because he always loved to eat.

Immediately I walked into my bedroom to be with Bruiser. "How is my trooper doing?" I asked while softly touching him. He meowed weakly, slowly lifted his head to look at me, calmly closed his eyes, and peacefully passed away.

Bruiser had waited to tell me goodbye and then quietly left me. I thought back to the time I first met him as a patient in the intensive care unit at the veterinary hospital and how no one expected him to find a home because he had feline AIDS. Yet, he had been my faithful friend for seven years. I will always remember him.

While Bruiser was with us, I also had several other cats. The chance of transmitting FIV from an infected cat to another is low. The disease is spread mostly through bite wounds. Bruiser was an easy-going peace lover. None of the other cats contracted feline AIDS even though they shared the same food and water dishes.

I hope that no one will terminate the precious life of a cat simply because they are FIV positive. They can provide several years of devoted companionship without transmitting the disease to other cats in the household. Presently a new vaccine has been approved to prevent feline AIDS. Hopefully it will lead the way for an HIV vaccine for humans.

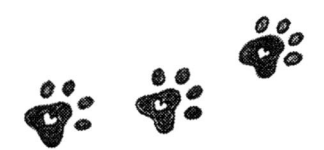

Dad seemed to be getting worse almost daily. Mom hired a home health care nurse to help bathe and take care of him. He had struggled with his disease for nearly sixteen years. The neurological specialists concluded that there was no treatment to stop or to reverse the degenerative process in his brain.

As a young, healthy, vibrant man, Dad fought proudly in World War II. He was a left rear tail gunner on a B-29 Super Fortress bomber and flew several missions over the Himalaya Mountains from India to China.

On one occasion he developed a severe inner ear infection and was hospitalized. While he was recovering, his outfit was sent on a bombing raid and they never returned. Dad was the only member to remain from his squadron. He received an honorable discharge and was sent home. Although his life was spared, the harsh inner ear infection possibly predisposed him to later degenerative brain lesions.

Every morning Dad would crawl out of bed, painfully lift himself into his wheelchair and slowly make his way into the kitchen. His first priority was to feed Pug. She patiently waited for him and then eagerly feasted upon her breakfast, while Dad slowly ate hot cereal. She seemed to enjoy her morning meals with him. Having Pug gave Dad something to live for.

Physically Dad's body was wearing out. Although he maintained a sharp mind, he wasn't able to readily communicate verbally. Sometimes people treated him as if he were mentally disabled, which angered me.

Dad had a legally written living will stating that he did not want artificial life support when that time arrived. I approached him about death. I asked him what he thought about euthanasia. I reminded him that as a veterinarian I had access to sodium pentobarbital, which was the controlled drug we used to euthanize animals. He began to cry. "No, you could lose your license," he slowly expressed.

After that I never mentioned the topic again. I graciously respect that even when he was in pain, miserable, and terminally ill, Dad thought about me first and my future. He did not want me to jeopardize what I had worked so long and hard for.

In February 1998, Dad developed an open sore on the bottom of his right foot. The sore would not heal. He also became extremely congested and struggled with increasing breathing difficulty.

Dad was admitted to the American Fork Hospital and was diagnosed with cellulitis and aspiration pneumonia. He remained hospitalized for several days. The doctor approached Mom about placing Dad in a care facility. "Many times the caregivers become physically exhausted and their health becomes jeopardized," he explained.

I respected Mom's needs as the primary caregiver and offered to help more and not work as much away from home. Instead of releasing Dad to the care center, we took him home. I had worked all night and shortly retired to bed after we got Dad settled in.

Soon afterwards I was abruptly wakened by a loud crash and Mom's uncontrollable screaming. I jumped out of bed to see what was wrong.

Dad had tried to use the toilet. To the end he remained proud and would not soil himself. Unfortunately, he was too weak to lower himself onto the toilet seat and fell, crashing onto the back of the reservoir. Water was spraying everywhere. Dad was lying in agonizing pain on the floor. Mom had now given up and was in tears.

I then realized that my wanting and expecting a good outcome for Dad at home wasn't helping either of them. I turned the water off from the toilet, helped dry Dad, and placed him in his wheelchair. Mom called the care center. They indicated that they were expecting him since the doctor had already spoken to them the day before.

Leaving Dad in the convalescent home was a

Farewell

gut-wrenching decision for mom and for me. But, as usual, Dad seemed to make the best of it. Actually, I think he enjoyed the daily physical therapy and nursing care. He always had an eye for pretty women and loved their attention.

The care center was only a block from our home. Every day Mom, Pug, and I would walk to the nursing home to visit. Pug was welcome inside the facilities and eagerly visited with the patients and staff on her way to and from dad's room.

Sometimes I would push Dad home in his wheelchair to watch basketball with us on television. We would enjoy some ice cream, soda pop, or hot chocolate together. We even went on daylong excursions. Perhaps the situation was best for everyone — I hoped.

In August Dad seemed to give up. He was frequently admitted to the hospital for aspiration pneumonia. The doctor strictly forbade him anything by mouth, and all of his nourishment was administered through the stomach tube. Physical therapy indicated that they could no longer help him. He mostly stayed in bed asleep.

On a Saturday morning I visited him. He had

difficulty breathing but refused to wear oxygen. When I patted him on the back, he coughed up some secretions and seemed to breathe more comfortably. Later that day, before going to work, I checked on him again and he was quietly sleeping.

My shift that day was to work straight through until Monday morning at the veterinary emergency clinic during the day, and at the human hospital during the night. Come Sunday night, about eight o'clock, my older brother Jim phoned me at work. "You better drive home now, Dad's not doing well. The doctor says he doesn't have much time."

Immediately I contacted my supervisor, Connie, and she allowed without hesitation, "Go."

Quickly I departed. The freeway entrance that I normally took to get home was closed that night due to road construction. Hurriedly, I tried to find another route and became hopelessly lost.

Finally I discovered another entrance and raced toward home. Suddenly a thunderstorm began to howl. The windshield wipers on the old Ford didn't work adequately, and I had difficulty seeing through the glaring and water-soaked windows. My frustration mounted as I worried that I wouldn't make it home to see Dad alive.

Finally, after all the desperation to quickly arrive home, I stopped fighting and just began to drive cautiously. "Dad was already gone," I felt. And I sensed a relief that he could be liberated from his misery.

When I arrived at the American Fork Hospital, the family was waiting for me. I was escorted into Dad's room to be with him. Jan, my niece, accompanied me.

"No tears," I thought, "only blessed relief."

On Sunday, August 30, 1998, at eight p.m. my father passed away. After struggling for several years, he died alone in the back of an ambulance while being transported from a care center to the hospital.

Again the self-proclaimed words, "No one should have to die alone," haunted me. "Please forgive me for not being with you," I mourned.

I argued the merciful need for physician-assisted euthanasia. "Terminally ill patients should be allowed the freedom to peacefully die surrounded by their loved ones at home, rather than to unknowingly struggle against death alone in a cold, sterile, impersonal environment."

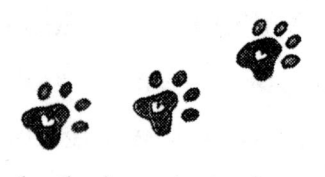

Dad and Mom had given me property behind their house and I built my home on it. After traveling the world and visiting its many wonders, I realized that my roots were firmly established at home in American Fork. That night Pug and I slept at Mom's house. I was used to Pug snuggling next to me, but she wasn't there. I got up and looked for her and discovered that she had crawled into bed with mom. The next morning Mom announced, "Guess who slept with me."

"I know, Mom, you needed an angel by your side last night."

"What a comfort the precious little thing was," Mom agreed.

That morning I took Pug to see Dad in his casket at the mortuary. I wanted her to know that she had seen him for the last time. I held her in my arms and she silently and motionlessly stared at him. Then we quietly left.

Farewell

Dad was buried in the American Fork Cemetery next to his dad and mom. He was given a military burial. Mom received the carefully folded American Flag.

In her eulogy Jan remembered her grandpa as the funny man who loved to work in his garden. Dad called a rose "one of life's greatest mysteries . . . the approach you take with it determines if it is beautiful, fragrant, and lovely — or ugly and thorny."

Jan recalled some of his favorite funny comments such as "Pass the sugar, sugar," or "We better jump into the water before it rains so we don't get wet." Jan also remembered some of the vacations we went on as a family. The simple things made Grandpa a hero to Jan.

Dad, may you be happy and joyful, walk briskly, and nurture your beautiful roses. And thanks for helping me to reach my goals. I know I was a pain sometimes. But you never gave up on me.

Farewell and love
Your son, Alan

Sleeping With Angels

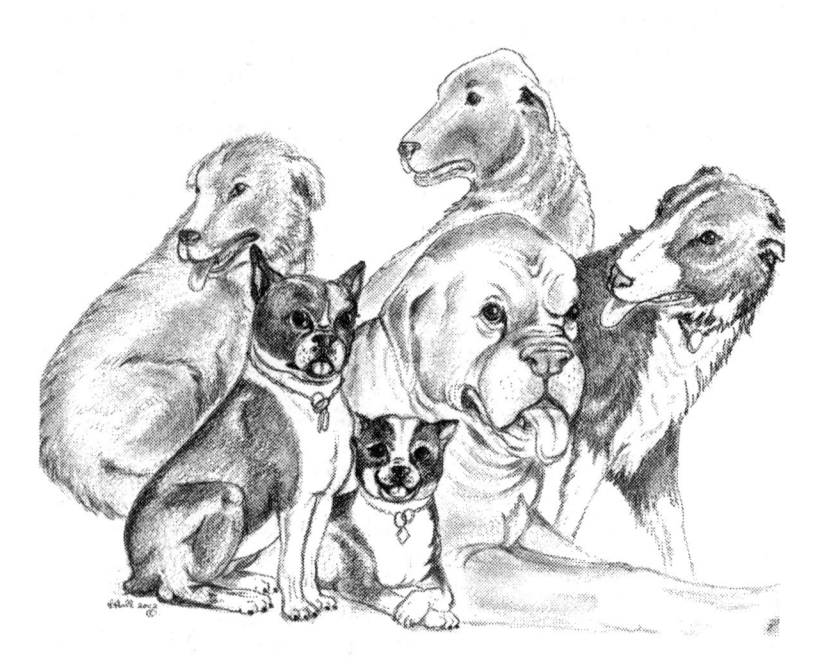

Legion of Angels

9
Unconditional Love

In late September 2000, in the early afternoon, I loaded all six of my dogs into the old 1969 green Ford. The Ford was now considered to be my "pet taxi." We traveled to Willow Park in the neighboring city of Lehi to go jogging on the Jordan River Parkway. I was training for the New York City Marathon to be held in November.

Shortly after obtaining Pug, my friends Clay and Joanie Robinson, former OSU classmates, had given me a Border Collie pup named Brownie. Since he was a herding dog, he loved to run and seemed to go forever without tiring. While Pug was the matriarch, Brownie was the peacemaker of the group. He was extremely sensitive, obedient, and intelligent.

Aspen was a three-legged Black Labrador. I

was working at the Utah Humane Society when she was admitted. As a young dog her left front leg had been severely broken and hung lifelessly at her side. When I first met her she seemed to beg for my attention and we quickly became friends.

The charge veterinarian suggested that I could amputate Aspen's useless leg in order to improve my surgical skills. Then, she added, we would either euthanize her, or try to arrange an adoption. Following the surgery Aspen awoke, looked at me, and wagged her tail. My heart was touched and I immediately felt obligated to take her home. She was the skeptical one.

Golden was a Golden Retriever. Someone had found him running loose on the street in front of the veterinary emergency clinic where I worked sometimes. He was apparently a homeless, stray pup. We accepted him into the clinic, and since he had no identification, we were obligated to notify the animal shelter. After one week no one claimed him. I took him home and discovered that he would be the rowdy one of the bunch.

C.C., my extremely friendly and outgoing dog, was a Boston Terrier pup. Her abbreviated name stood for chew, chew, chew, chewy, which didn't seem appropriate — so I shortened it to C.C. Amy, a veterinary technician, recognized my special love for Bostons, and gave her to me. She heard of a family in a homeless shelter that had her and couldn't keep her with them. Amy placed a ribbon and bow around C.C.'s neck and presented her to me as a Christmas gift.

Finally Moose, the shy one. He was a Neapolitan Mastiff. His owner and breeder wasn't able to sell him as a pup because he had an umbilical hernia. She offered him to me and of course I said, "I've always wanted a giant breed dog."

"Mom, guess what I have," I mentioned before introducing Moose to her.

"I hope it's not another dog," she warned.

I prudently brought Moose into the house and stood him on the living room floor to show him to mom. Immediately he nervously began to urinate. Mom had just cleaned the carpet. Needless to say, me and the six dogs had to escape on a road trip for a couple of days until things settled down at home.

"No more dogs," was the greeting I received

Sleeping With Angels

when we arrived home. Then Mom quickly softened and asked, "How was your trip, were the dogs okay?"

"Yes," I said. I didn't tell her how difficult it was to sneak six dogs into a motel room.

Besides the dogs I possessed many other wonderful animals: twenty cats, three love birds, one skunk, two raccoons, an ever-changing number of chickens and doves, one duck, two geese, two peacocks, and one wild turkey that aspired to be a chicken in drag.

If something needed a home, I would provide. My animals were my family and I loved and protected them as if they were my own children. Of course, the dogs were my closest companions.

All of them were well taken care of. Mom and I made sure of it. And, if you wonder, our yards received several beautification awards. Moreover, my log home was boasted to be like a page from "Better Homes and Gardens."

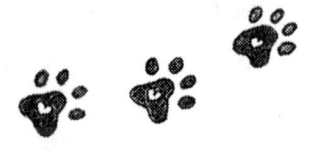

Returning to the marathon training: Since all six

dogs were with me, I decided to go on a shorter three mile run with them rather than a longer run. Brownie was designated my long run partner, sometimes up to twenty miles. Aspen, being three-legged, tired easily, although she was determined to forge ahead with us one difficult step at a time. Moose, whose legs were monstrously large, tended to drag his feet after awhile and to wear off his bottom pads.

Pug, as usual, had her own agenda. Mom often claimed, "Pug isn't a dog, she's a person." Sometimes I agreed with her.

Pug had jogging figured out. "What nonsense, I would rather explore," she seemed to debate. Besides, densely vegetated riverbanks provided a kaleidoscope of adventures for her.

"For now that's okay. We'll be back soon," I told her.

Upon returning, Pug was nowhere to be found. "Pug," I called. No answer. Immediately we retraced our steps. "Perhaps she decided to follow us." Still no Pug. "Could she be waiting at the car?"

"Pug," I again called. She wasn't there.

Frantically I yelled for her. I fiercely blamed

myself for leaving her alone. "Pug was too smart to get into trouble or to let anyone take her," I tried to reason.

Again we retraced our steps. I asked people in the campsites if they had noticed her. They all answered that they hadn't. I stopped at the park manager's but he wasn't there. I placed a note on his door describing Pug and about when she was lost. I then added my name, phone number, and address.

I worried that the animal control officer might have seen her running loose and picked her up.

Distraught, we returned home without Pug. None of the animal shelters I called knew anything of her.

"Where's Pug?" Mom alarmingly asked when we returned home.

"I'm afraid I don't know. We went jogging and she didn't follow us. When we returned I couldn't find her." Without warning my floodgates opened wide and I sobbed so hard I could barely breathe.

"Let's go look again," Mom rationally suggested.

Repeatedly we searched for Pug, but with no success. We called loudly, "Pug, Pug!" I brought C.C. and Brownie with us for their help, but still we couldn't locate her. Devastated, we again returned home without Pug.

Nearly five hours had passed. Nightfall was quickly approaching. "I must continue searching for her."

Mom would stay home to listen for any phone calls. Pug wore an identification tag on her collar. We prayed someone would call.

Brownie, C.C., and I again drove back to Willow Park. On our way there I noticed a father with his young daughter. They were driving in a black Ford Ranger truck. In the truck bed was a Boston Terrier freely pacing back and forth, from side to side. In my confused mind I thought it was Pug. Quickly I followed the vehicle. Shortly it stopped and I eagerly approached the young driver. I thought for sure he had taken Pug. But when I looked more closely I realized it wasn't her. "Sorry," I apologized. "I just lost my Boston Terrier and I mistook yours for her. Again, I'm so sorry," I said with unmasked emotion.

He seemed sensitive to my needs and replied, "I hope you find her."

We soon arrived back at Willow Park. Determined to find her, we searched everywhere for Pug. But, no success. I stopped at the park manager's a second time. This time he was present. He said that it was his day off and normally he wouldn't have been there. I asked him if he had seen a Boston Terrier. "I lost her around noon," I explained.

"Are you Alan Cunningham?" he asked.

"Yes," I anxiously replied.

"Boy, are you in luck. A younger gentleman just left from here. He has your dog in the front seat of his truck. He noticed your name and address on her tags and is taking her to your house. I saw the note you left on my door earlier today and told him that you had lost her. You just missed him."

The park manager continued, "The man said that he was in his boat fishing when he noticed a little dog in the water. She was struggling to get out but the riverbank was so steep that she would temporarily cling at the loose dirt embankment and then repeatedly fall back into the river. She kept struggling like this with no success. Fortunately, she was able to climb onto a large tree limb extending over the water. This allowed her to stay afloat and to rest."

"Thank you," I sighed with relief. Immediately we drove home. Nearly seven hours had elapsed. I wondered how long Pug had actually struggled in the cold, murky water. "Probably most of the time," I ghastly speculated. Thankfully, the fisherman had seen and rescued her.

When I drove into Mom's driveway she was outside holding Pug, wrapped in a warm blanket. She said the fisherman had dried her off, worried that she was cold and in shock. Relief swept over me.

"Here's your baby," Mom consoled.

Mom gently handed an exhausted Pug over to me.

"The man who returned her just left."

"Did you get his name?" I asked. I wanted to call and thank him.

"No, he didn't tell me his name. And I was so excited to have Pug back that I never thought to ask."

Sleeping With Angels

Pug must have had a guardian angel watching over her that day, I decided.

"Thank you, whoever you are. Thank you, Thank you, Thank you."

"Pug knew that you wouldn't give up on her. She could probably hear you calling for her throughout the afternoon," Mom sympathized.

"She loved you so much that she refused to give up as well. Unconditional love grows even stronger when it is reciprocated."

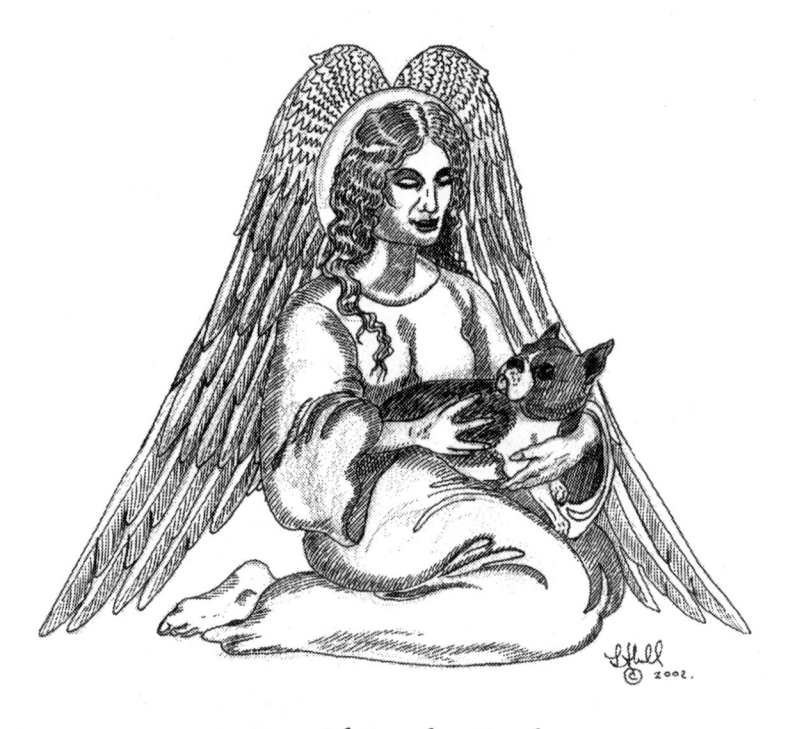

Pug with Guardian Angel

10
A Breath Away

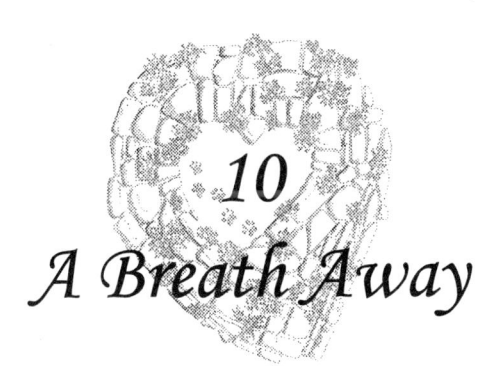

Yes, Pug was the matriarch. She tolerated no nonsense from the other dogs. She and C.C. stayed in the house while the larger dogs remained outside. Although my house was next door to mom's, we spent most of our time with mom in her home. She enjoyed our company and we hers.

Pug, as is common with Boston Terriers, was also fearless. She would readily take on any challenge. If a stray dog entered the yard, no matter the size, she would quickly send it on its way. She became totally focused on her crusade of keeping unwanted animal intruders away. Oftentimes she would carelessly run in front of cars as she chased after the unwelcome visitors.

One early July morning Pug determined to chase after another dog across the street. Boldly

Sleeping With Angels

and recklessly she ran in front of a car in her attempt to scare off the other dog. The oncoming elderly driver couldn't stop fast enough. Pug limped away and the driver continued on. Mom noticed her waiting on the porch and let her in the house. She hobbled into my bedroom, not placing weight on her right rear leg, and stared up at me with helpless eyes.

"What's wrong, little girl," I asked. I noticed she wasn't using her leg. I palpated it, and the upper portion of her femur felt unstable.

"Mom," I called, "do you know what happened to Pug? She's not using her back leg, I think it's broken."

"No," she answered, "I let her out to use the bathroom and when I let her back in she was limping."

Later we were informed by a witnessing neighbor of what had happened.

"Don't you think you better take her to the veterinarian," Mom asked.

"Ouch," I flinched. I bit my tongue momentarily and then chuckled to myself. Mom carelessly had a habit of making that statement whenever my animals needed veterinary care.

"I'll take her to the emergency clinic," I consented. Occasionally I did relief veterinary work at Animal Emergency South.

Radiographs revealed a comminuted (fragmented) fracture in the proximal portion of her right femur. Pug would need orthopedic surgery. I didn't have the expertise or experience to confidently approach the necessary procedure. So I called the Roy Veterinary Clinic. Dr. Pearson, Dr. Talbot, and Dr. Moss, whom I consider to be excellent veterinarians and my mentors, were on staff. Dr. Pearson said that he would be happy to repair Pug's leg.

I trusted Pug would be in good care. But when I left her at the hospital she looked at me with large, questioning eyes. My heart melted. "I'll be back."

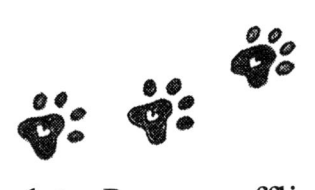

Nearly one year later Pug was afflicted with medical problems in her right front leg.

"Alan, come here quick, something's wrong with Pug," Mom called.

I was outside with the other dogs but quickly answered Mom's request. Pug was painfully holding up her right front leg, her eyes full of agony.

"What's wrong, Pug?" I checked her leg but could feel no instability. Neither could I feel any foreign bodies such as thorns or puncture weeds. "Did you sprain your wrist," I consoled.

"I don't think it's broken. Perhaps she sprained or bruised it."

I then gave Pug a non-steroidal anti-inflammatory called rimadyl. Later on, when she should have been feeling better, she still appeared to be in extreme pain. "Perhaps she has a fracture or a torn ligament or tendon," I reasoned.

Again I took her to the emergency center where I had recently started working full-time. Radiographs revealed "significant arthritis but no fractures, or dislocations," Dr. Anderson critiqued. I then gave her torbugesic, which was a more potent pain medication than rimadyl.

Still Pug appeared terribly uncomfortable. The next day, after a sleepless night, we returned to the emergency clinic. Dr. Howell, who was on staff, checked Pug. "Do you feel how cold her foot is," she observed.

"Yes," I agreed.

"I wonder if she has a blood clot? Let's give her an injection of heparin," she advised. "And we'll also change her pain medication to buprenex, it should work more effectively."

That night, while I was working as a respiratory therapist in the hospital emergency room, I approached the E. R. physician about Pug's symptoms. Dr. Supranowicz suggested an ultrasound to rule out blood clots. I then called Dr. Watkins, the veterinary internal medicine specialist. He promised, "I'll see you tomorrow at ten a.m. at the emergency clinic."

The next morning arrived. The doppler showed no blood flow in Pug's entire right front leg. The ultrasound indicated a clot in the armpit or axillary region somewhere between the subclavian artery and the axillary artery. Dr. Watkins advised intravenous fluids, heparin therapy, strong pain medication, and hospitalization.

"I'm very sorry," he comforted. Then he cautioned, "I'm afraid she might lose her leg."

"Thanks for your help," I somberly replied. "Good luck."

I quietly picked up Pug and walked outside to grieve. Due to severe arthritis from her previous fracture, Pug seldom used her back leg. What would she do now without the front leg? I selfishly refused to entertain euthanasia as an option; she still had too much life ahead of her.

After some private time together I resolved to vigorously attack the problem. With the help of the technicians, we started IV fluids, heparin therapy, and ran blood tests. Also, we placed a fentanyl patch snugly across the back of her neck for continuous pain relief. And of course, Pug returned home with me for her ongoing medical care.

Slowly she began to improve. With the exception of her foot, the rest of her leg became warm with restored circulation. Miraculously we had saved her leg.

Because of the initial compromised blood flow in Pug's leg, the tissue died and sloughed from her foot, leaving the bones exposed in her wrist and toes. Daily we soaked her foot and changed the dressing. Our hope was that by removing the decaying flesh, new and healthy tissue could replace it.

Through all this Pug was a champion. Although she hurt, she never complained. I believed that she was getting better and that I had my old Pug back.

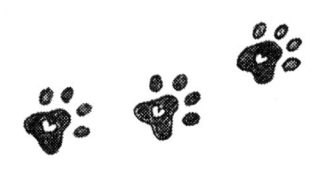

Pug and C.C. often accompanied me to work at the veterinary clinic. Besides their companionship, it allowed me to more effectively treat Pug's leg. On Sunday, August 11, 2002, we were working at the hospital. There I have my own office and bedroom to rest in when things are quiet. Pug, C.C., and I were sleeping together. Around five a.m. Pug woke up and looked over the side of the bed at her food and water dishes.

"Are you thirsty, little girl?" I helped her down and she drank. "Lets go outside to the bathroom, you two." I carried Pug, and C.C. followed. I placed Pug on the grass. Tiny step by step, she slowly limped a short way, and then quietly sat down. When I called her to come back she acted

Sleeping With Angels

as if she couldn't hear me. I gently picked her up and we returned to the bedroom. When I placed Pug on the bed she began breathing laboriously. I noticed that her gums were pale and felt cold to touch. Suddenly, without warning, she collapsed.

Immediately I gathered her in my arms.

"Shannan," I called. "Can you help me?"

Shannan was asleep in the technician's bedroom "What's wrong?" she asked with concern.

"Pug's dying," I sobbed.

"What do you want me to do, Dr. Cunningham?" she quietly inquired.

"I don't want Pug to suffer anymore. Can you get the euthanasia solution?"

Before Shannan could obtain the drug Pug passed away. I collapsed to the floor with her in my arms.

"Oh Pug," I cried. "Why did you leave me?"

"You did the best you could for her, Dr. Cunningham," Shannan expressed with sympathy. "Maybe she had another blood clot."

After a few moments she said, "You know, be grateful that she went quickly and didn't suffer."

Through Shannan's practical advice I felt somewhat comforted. Thankfully I realized that Pug had awakened me to tell me goodbye one last time.

"Let me wrap her in a blanket. When you feel ready you can take her home," Shannan offered.

C.C. waited patiently. Usually she competed with Pug for my attention. But now she simply stood back and silently watched. I gathered my things and carried C.C. out to the truck. I then cradled Pug into my arms. We slowly drove home with her in my lap. I remembered this was how I carried her home eleven years before as a pup, curled up in my lap.

When I arrived home, Mom was still asleep. I entered her bedroom with Pug in my arms and began to sob uncontrollably.

"What's wrong?" Mom asked with alarm.

"Pug's gone."

Mom began to cry. "You've known from the start that she wasn't going to make it, didn't you?"

"Yes," I nodded.

"You were able to be with her when she died and that's what you wanted."

Sleeping With Angels

"Yes," I again nodded.

"Pug's with Dad now. They can both run and play together. She is much happier."

I gently placed Pug on her bed. She looked so peaceful. One more time I wished to sleep with my angel next to me.

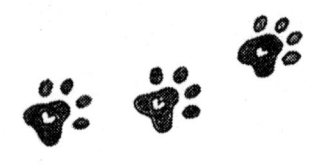

I could not bury my little girl. Finally I phoned my cousin Kathy, a genuine animal lover. Without hesitation she offered, "We'll be right there."

Pug was still wrapped in the covering Shannan had placed around her.

I gathered my five other dogs. One by one they sniffed her and said goodbye. Then I carefully placed Pug in the grave I had dug. Tenderly I arranged her to make sure she wasn't resting on her injured legs. One last time I caressed her and then smoothed and tucked the blanket around her. Kathy's husband Peter buried Pug for me. With great care and respect he covered her tiny body with earth. Kathy then offered a prayer.

I had chosen a special location just for Pug

under the flowering crab apple tree between my house and mom's house. She often loved to escape by herself and rest in the shade outside when it was hot. I placed her adjacent to a white concrete bench. On the bench was a statue of a boy and his dog sitting by each other. I also rested a sandstone boulder on the ground above her. I had found this stone on the last outing my six dogs and I had taken to Southern Utah.

The next morning I discovered a freshly cut rose on Pug's grave. Mom had placed it there. And she continues to visit Pug's grave and talk to her.

Pug was gone. I felt immense emptiness. My beloved companion had died about one week before her eleventh birthday and four years after Dad's passing. They both died on a Sunday.

"God," I pleaded, "please comfort me. Let me know Pug is all right."

That night I dreamed of Pug dancing happily in a beautiful meadow. She was joyously accompanied by my father who was playing with her.

Dad had loaned Pug to me for a short time. I had given her to him some eleven years earlier. Now it was his turn to have her back.

Even though she was gone Pug, in her unconditional and unselfish love, had painstakingly prepared for me a legion of angels — namely C.C., Brownie, Golden, Aspen, and Moose. Pug had slept by my side, as my angel, up to the moment she passed away. Briefly she woke to say one last goodbye and then quietly left.

During her short and precious life, Pug had faithfully escorted me — one diligent step at a time — from veterinary school graduation to an established profession as a licensed veterinarian.

I dearly miss you, Pug. You are my angel and forever love. You will never be absent from my heart.

"And know you're there, a breath away's not far to where you are."

From the song "To Where You Are" by Josh Groban and Richard Marx

A Breath Away

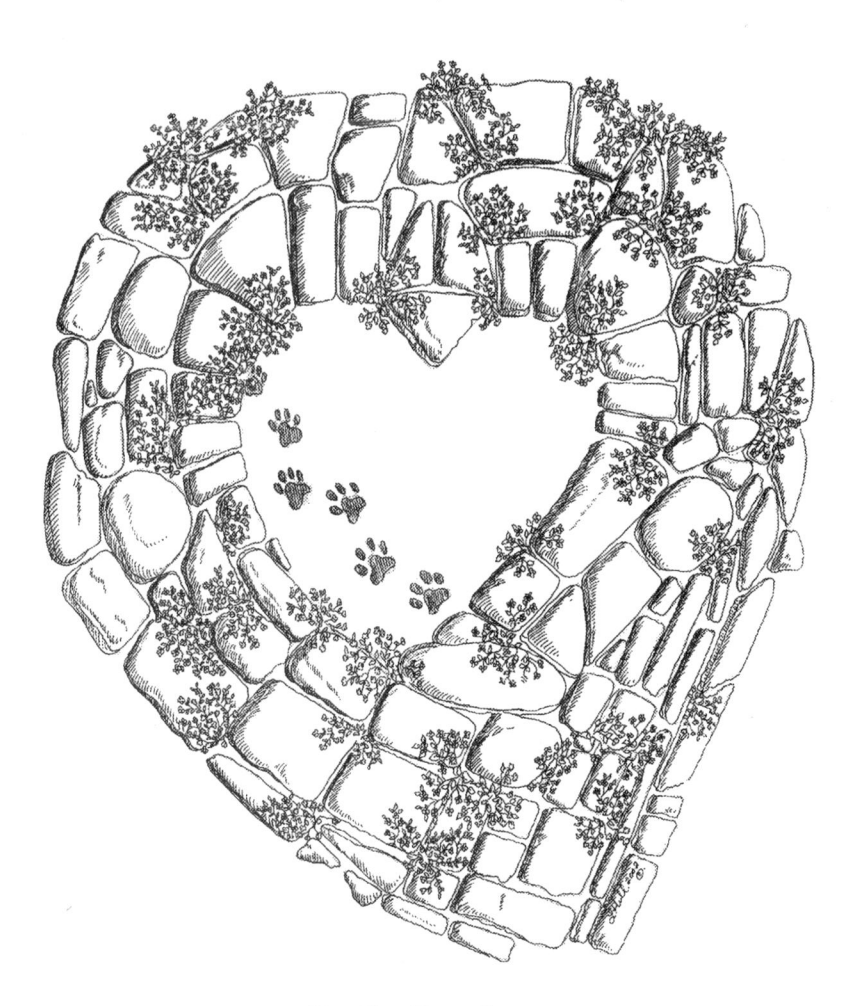

Stepping Stone Journey

Rainbow Bridge

Just this side of heaven is a place called Rainbow Bridge. When an animal dies who has been especially close to someone here, that pet goes to Rainbow Bridge. There are meadows and hills for all of our special friends so they can run and play together. There is plenty of food and water, and sunshine, and our friends are warm and comfortable.

All the animals who have been ill or old are restored to health and vigor, those who were hurt or maimed are made whole and strong again, just as we remember them in our dreams of days and time gone by. The animals are happy and content, except for one small thing; each one misses someone very special who had been left behind.

They all run and play together, but the day comes when one suddenly stops and looks into the distance. His bright eyes are intent; his eager body begins to quiver. All at once he begins to run from the group, flying over the green grass, his legs carrying him faster and faster.

A Breath Away

You have been spotted, and when you and your special friend finally meet you cling together in joyous reunion, never to be parted again. The happy kisses rain upon your face; your hands again caress the beloved head, and you look once more into the trusting eyes of your pet, so long gone from your life but never absent from you heart.

Then you cross Rainbow Bridge together...
Author Unknown

Sleeping With Angels

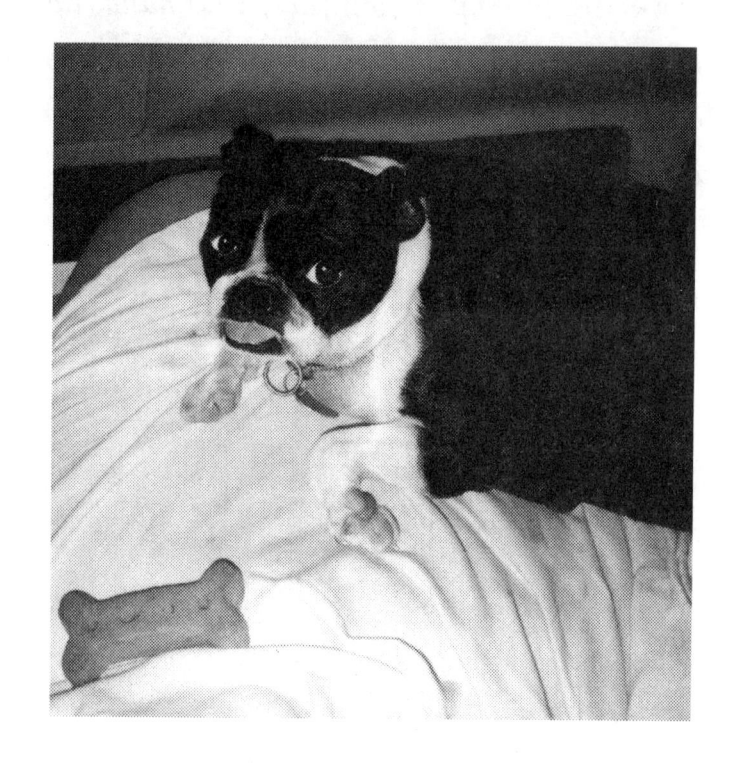

In Memory
Pug
August 21, 1991 to August 11, 2002

About the Author

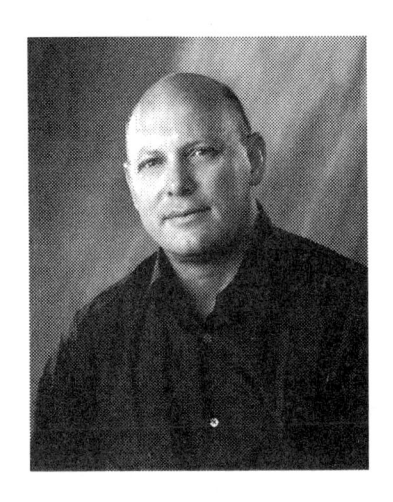

Dr. Alan B. Cunningham graduated from Brigham Young University with a Bachelor of Science in Animal Science and a Masters Degree in Respiratory Health Care Science. He also graduated from Utah State University with a Ph.D. in physiology and later from Oregon State University with a Doctorate in Veterinary Medicine.

Presently Dr. Cunningham is one of twenty worldwide veterinarians selected to participate in the flexible Medical Curriculum for Professionals Program, leading to a Doctor of Medicine Degree at the University of Health Sciences Antigua. This unique program recognizes the significant bond between human and veterinary medicine and emphasizes training doctors toward strengthening that relationship.

He is also the recipient of the Wilfred O. Foundation Scholarship. In return, after graduating from medical school, he will be providing medical and veterinary services to rural and medically underserved areas of the world.

Dr. Cunningham is a strong supporter of people-pet rehabilitation. Furthermore he campaigns for a national monument to be erected for animals that have served our country as valiant wartime soldiers. In addition to advocating physician-assisted euthanasia for the terminally ill, he also promotes public school education to youth about birth control and sexually transmitted diseases.

Aside from the companionship with his beloved animals, Dr. Cunningham enjoys gardening, traveling, running marathons, and oil painting. He is

About the Author

an avid fan of Cirque du Soleil. He considers visiting the natural and man-made wonders of the world as one of his most worthwhile achievements. Furthermore, he recalls working as a volunteer in the 2002 Winter Olympics in Salt Lake City as a memorable experience.

In addition to attending medical school, Dr. Cunningham currently works as a licensed veterinarian at a nighttime emergency clinic, and also as a registered respiratory therapist for Intermountain Health Care. He is a lifelong resident of American Fork, Utah.

*"To every thing there is a season, and
a time to every purpose under the heaven:
A time to be born, and a time to die…
A time to weep, and a time to laugh…
a time to keep silence, and a time to speak…"*
                                    Ecclesiastes 3:1-7